Restoring
Natural Harmony

天
人
合
一

Simon Blow

First published 2010
Copyright © 2010 Simon Blow

National Library of Australia
Cataloguing-in-Publication data:

Simon Blow

Restoring Natural Harmony

ISBN: 978-0-9873417-5-4

Published by:
The Genuine Wisdom Centre
PO Box 446
Summer Hill NSW 2130
Australia
(www.genuinewisdomcentre.com)

Editing:
Essence Writing (www.essencewriting.com.au)

Cover design and layout:
Determind Design (www.determind.com.au)

Diagrams:
John Bennetts

Disclaimer
The intention of this book is to present information and practices that have been used throughout China for many years. The information offered is according to the author's best knowledge and is to be used by the reader at his or her own discretion and liability. Readers should obtain professional advice where appropriate regarding their health and health practices. The author disclaims all responsibility and liability to any person, arising directly or indirectly from taking or not taking action based upon the information in this publication.

This book is dedicated to

… all those lovers of peace

Contents

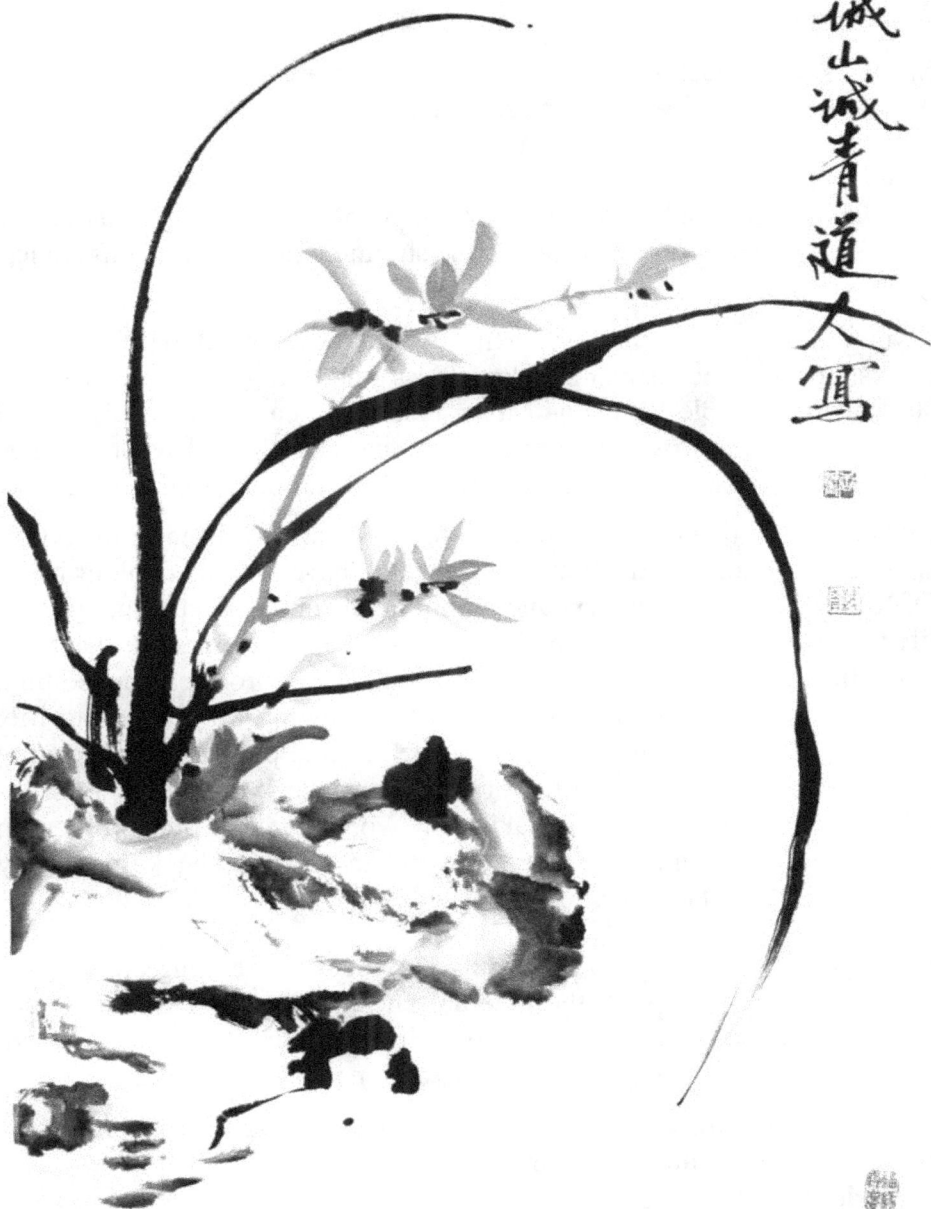

青城山诚青道大写

Mountain Orchid by Taoist Priest Grand Master Tang, Qing Cheng Shan
Green City Mountain, China. September 2004

Acknowledgements

There are many people I would like to thank for helping me to compile and develop this book.

Since I started teaching full-time in 1992, I have taught 18 to 22 classes per week – the best way to learn something is to teach it, as the old saying goes. This is especially relevant when working with the universal life force Qi energy, as it is important to be in front of people to share this energy. Qigong Master Jack Lim told me that when you are teaching a class, think of it as being with a group of friends and sharing. Thank you for this advice, Jack.

I would like to thank all those friends who have attended my classes and workshops over the years. I get many ideas and positive feedback from the students and people I meet and from those who have generously shared their own experiences. I'm not sure if we have original ideas or if, when the heart opens and the Qi flows, we are simply all one. Again, thank you.

I would like to thank Dr Xu Hongtao for his guidance, friendship and for sharing the Qigong cultivation practices that I have presented in this book. Dr Xu has a very deep understanding of Qigong and Guigen Qigong is his life's passion and I feel privileged that I have the opportunity to share this with others. I would like to thank Lynn Guilhaus for proofreading, editing, researching and additional writing and for bringing this project to life. I'm also grateful to John Bennetts for the original photos and adaptation to drawings; they are all works of art. Thank you to Adriene Hurst for her persistence in editing and making my words come to life and Mamun Khan from Determind Design for the layout and design. Thanks also to my friends at NPT Offset Press.

We refer to Qigong as an art form. It is a process of refining our internal energy to harmonise with the external energy or environment. It's our own observation of our relationship with everything around us. We are influenced by everything around us, we are one with everything.

I have had the fortunate opportunity to meet many great masters, professors and doctors, but mainly, just great people who are committed to contributing to the development of the human race. Thank you.

About the Author: Simon Blow

A near-fatal accident at the age of nineteen lead Simon to investigate various methods of healing and rejuvenation, a path he has been following ever since. Simon is a Sydney-based (Australia) master teacher (Laoshi) of the ancient Chinese art of longevity and has been leading regular classes for beginning and continuing students since 1990.

Having travelled the world to learn and explore this ancient art, Simon has received extensive training and certification from many respected sources: Traditional Chinese Medical Hospitals and Daoist Monasteries in China, Buddhist Monasteries in Australia, and Hindu Ashrams in India. He has been given authority to share these techniques through his teachings and publications.

Simon received World Health Organisation Certification in Medical Qigong clinical practice from the Xiyuan Hospital in Beijing and is a Standing Council Member of the World Academic Society of Medical Qigong in Beijing. He has also been initiated into Dragon Gate Daoism and given the name of Xin Si, meaning Genuine Wisdom.

His dedication, compassion and wisdom also make Simon a sought-after keynote speaker and workshop facilitator. By demand he has created a series of Book/DVD sets and guided meditation CDs. He also helps produce CDs for the Sunnatram Forest Monastery, the YWCA Encore program and a series of Meditation CDs for children and teenagers.

China holds a special place in Simon's heart. He has had the great fortune to travel to China on many occasions to study Qigong, attend international conferences, tour the sacred mountains and experience the rich couture of the Chinese people. Since 1999 he has been leading unique study tours to China so he could take people to the source and give them the opportunity to experience first-hand this ancient healing practice.

Romanisation of Chinese words

The Genuine Wisdom Centre uses the Pinyin romanisation system of Chinese to English. Pinyin is a name for the system used to transliterate Chinese words into the Roman alphabet. The use of Pinyin was first adopted in the 1950s by the Chinese government, and it became official in 1979 when it was endorsed by the People's Republic of China.

Pinyin is now standard in the People's Republic of China and in several world organisations, including the United Nations. Pinyin replaces the Wade-Giles and Yale systems.

Some common conversions:

Pinyin	Also spelled as	Pronunciation
Qi	Chi	Chee
Qigong	Chi Kung	Chee Kung
Taiji	Tai Chi	Tai Jee
Taijiquan	Tai Chi Chuan	Tai Jee Chuen
Gongfu	Kung Fu	Gong Foo
Dao	Tao	Dao
Daoism	Taoism	Daoism
Dao De Jing	Tao Teh Ching	Dao Teh Ching

How to use this book

Traditionally we follow the teacher/master and this balances our energy. The book gives detailed instructions on how to perform the movements and provides additional theory and history to complement the practises. To view videos showing the shape of the movements please visit our YouTube channel
www.yoututbe.com/simonblowqigong

It's important to learn from an experienced qualified teacher and to practise regularly to master the movements yourself. Attending regular classes provides consistent practice and refinement and the energy of the group nurtures and supports everyone. It's important not to stray too far from the flock.

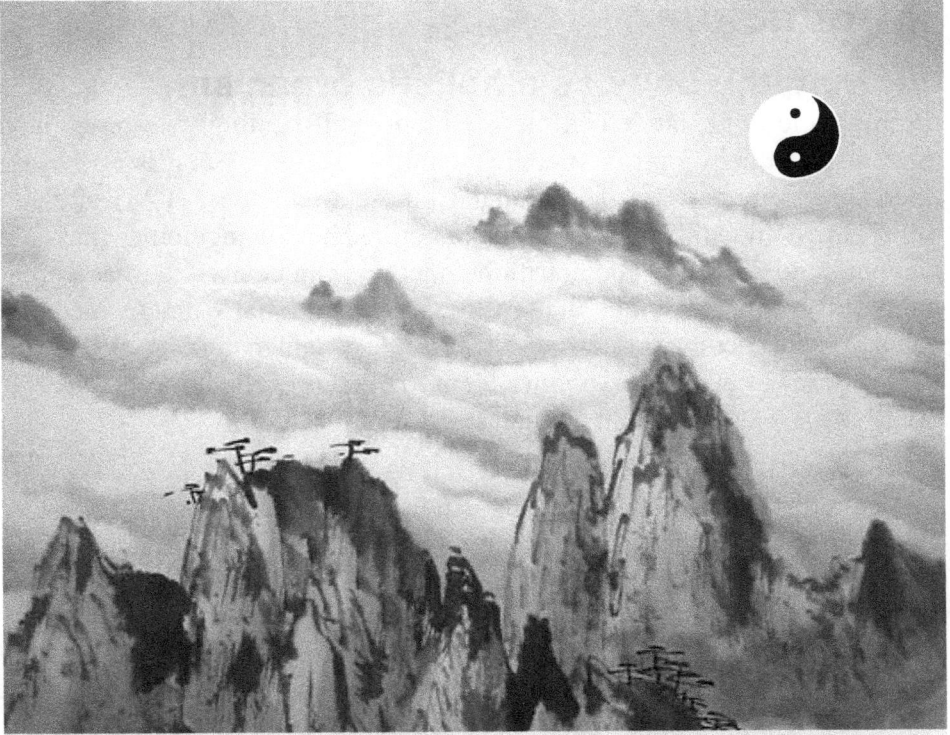

Chapter 1

Introduction

Restoring Natural Harmony

Introduction

Viewing the body as a holistic organism

From ancient to modern times, Qigong self-healing exercises have been used to help improve people's quality of life. Qigong is one of the therapeutic methods of Traditional Chinese Medicine (TCM) and like other TCM modalities such as acupuncture, herbal medicine, massage, cupping, moxibustion, and nutritional therapy, can be used to treat a broad range of both chronic and acute illnesses. Traditional Chinese medicine is an ancient medical system that takes a deep understanding of the laws and patterns of nature and applies them to the human body. At the heart of TCM is Qi – the force that animates and informs all things.

Traditional Chinese Medicine

An important principle underlying Traditional Chinese Medicine (TCM) is the understanding of the balance and harmony between human beings and our environment. Daoism and TCM view the human being as a micro (internal) representation of our macro (external) environment. It is based on the concept that the human body is a small universe with a set of complete and sophisticated interconnected systems, and that those systems usually work in balance and with the forces of nature to maintain the healthy function of the human body. TCM seeks to heal the root causes of dysfunction or disease and has been practised for over 5,000 years, making it one of the oldest and most widely used systems of medicine in the world.

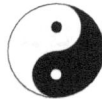

In this ancient vision of the body, the internal organs function differently from the way they are understood to function in Western Medicine. Unlike the Western medical model which divides the physical body into anatomical structures, the Chinese model is more concerned with function. Thus, the TCM heart is not a specific piece of flesh, but an aspect of function related to consciousness, mental vitality and unclouded thinking.

Each solid organ (Yin) has a corresponding flowing organ (Yang). TCM understands that everything is composed of two complementary energies; one energy is Yin and the other is Yang. They are never separate; one cannot exist without the other. This relationship is reflected in the black and white Yin/Yang symbol. No matter how you try to divide this circle in half, each section will always contain both energies.

The organs also correspond to the Five Elements, relating to different seasons, colours and emotions. The belief that the human body is a microcosm of the Universal macrocosm means that humans must follow the laws of the Universe to achieve harmony and total health. The Yin/Yang and Five-Element theories are observations and descriptions of Universal law, not concepts created by man. These essential theories form the basis of TCM and are used today to understand, diagnose and treat health problems. The network of relationships is complex, and scholars study and meditate for many years to fully understand these connections between the internal and the external world.

According to Taoist Master Hua-Ching Ni:

"Chi is the vital universal energy which composes, permeates and moves everything that exists. Chi may be defined as the ultimate cause, and at the same time, as the ultimate effect. Chi is the ultimate essence of the universe as well as the law of all movement. When Chi conglomerates, it is called matter. When Chi is diffuse, it is called space. When Chi animates form, it is called life. When Chi separates and withdraws from form, it is called death. When Chi flows, there is health. When Chi is blocked, there is sickness and disease. Chi embraces all things, circulates through and sustains them. The planets depend on it for their brightness, weather is formed by it, and the seasons are caused by it. So it is Chi, or vital energy, which activates and maintains all life. Chi animates all processes of the body: the digestion and assimilation of the food we eat, the inhalation and exhalation of air by the lungs, the circulation of the blood, the dissemination of fluids throughout the body and, finally, the excretion of waste products of the metabolism.

"The Yellow Emperor's Internal Canon of Medicine in 2,500BC explains, "One is able to smell only if the lung Qi penetrates to the nose. One can distinguish the five colours only if the liver Qi penetrates to the eyes. One can hear only if the kidney Qi penetrates the ears. One can taste only if the heart Qi penetrates the tongue. One can know whether food is palatable only if the spleen Qi penetrates the mouth. The capabilities of the seven orifices depend upon the penetration of Qi from the five solid organs."

When I was studying Guigen Qigong with Dr Xu at the Xiyuan Hospital in Beijing, I asked him if I also needed to study TCM. "No," he answered, "It would put too much information in your mind. It's better to understand the basic principle." Similarly, while it's good to know how your car works, you don't need a degree in mechanical engineering to maintain and service your car.

The Five Element Theory

In 'Book 1 - The Art of Life', I introduced The Five Element Qigong Meditation and the Five Element Theory – an ancient understanding of the natural world, it's movement and transformation. We as human beings are also an integral part of this system. This theory, together with the theory of Yin and Yang, are the main methods used in Traditional Chinese Medicine and Daoism to help explain our connection to and relationship with our environment and the universe.

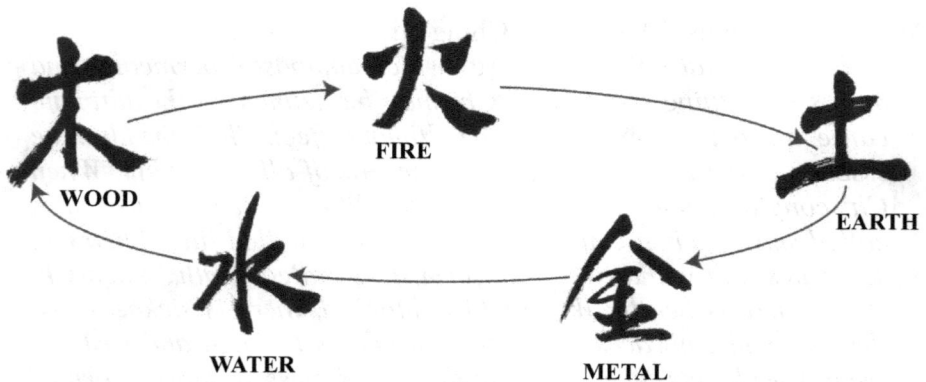

	EARTH	METAL	WATER	WOOD	FIRE
Zang Organ (Yin)	Spleen	Lungs	Kidneys	Liver	Heart
Fu organ (Yang)	Stomach	Large Intestine	Urinary Bladder	Gall Bladder	Small Intestine
Season	Late summer	Autumn	Winter	Spring	Summer
Plant part	Fruit	Compost	Seed	Shoot	Flower
Function	Harvest	Death	Storing	Sprouting	Blossoming
Emotion	Worry	Grief	Fear	Anger	Joy/ Excitement
Colour	Yellow	White	Deep Blue/ black	Green	Red
Type of Qi	Dampness	Dryness	Cold	Wind	Heat

The theory of the five elements says that all things in the natural world are derived from wood, fire, earth, metal and water. The elements all possess specific properties and are related to each other and act on each other. The order of generation among the five elements is that water generates wood, wood generates fire, fire generates earth, earth generates metal, and metal generates water. In this way generation is circular and endless. The way to remember this is to follow the natural order of the seasons: the Spleen (late Summer), Lungs (Autumn) Kidneys (Winter), Liver (Spring), and Heart (Summer).

Meridians

Meridians are pathways or channels which transport Qi and blood through the whole body ensuring the tissues and organs are supplied with fluids and nutrients. They are all interconnected with each other and form a network helping connect the internal organs (Five Elements) to external parts of the body. Good health is a result of Qi flowing smoothly through the meridian system. Diseases, physical and emotional problems can occur when this system is blocked or impeded.

The art of Qigong consists of meditation, relaxation, physical movement, mind-body integration and breathing exercises. Qigong describes all the Chinese energy or Qi techniques that promote the flow of Qi through the energy channels of the body and connects the body with the energy of the universe. If practised regularly, Qigong can promote calmness of mind, vitality, good health and spiritual awareness.

When our mind is at peace our Qi flows smoothly creating harmony with the universe.

"Too much colour, the eyes cannot enjoy.
Too much noise, the ears cannot receive, and music cannot be heard or appreciated.
Too complicated, too prepared, or too processed food causes the tongue to lose its taste.
Too much rushing around, hunting and searching, maddens the mind.
Too much interest in hard-to-obtain goods distorts one's behaviour.
The wise one likes to maintain one's inner essence, and thus is not enslaved by sensory pleasure.
Sensory pleasures and the outer search for material goods create burdens and cause one's life to become scattered."
Lao Tzu, Dao De Jing, Chapter 12

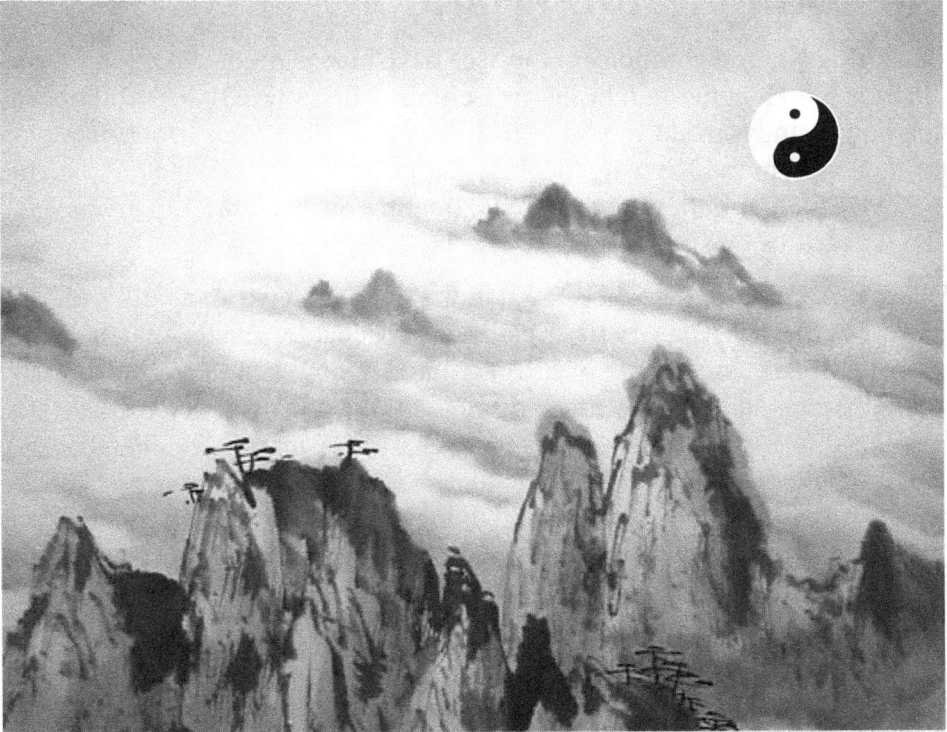

Chapter 2

Restoring Natural Harmony

Restoring Natural Harmony

Restoring Natural Harmony

Restoring Natural Harmony comprises the Chinese Medical Qigong forms that Dr Xu Hongtao taught me in Beijing. I first met Dr Xu while I was leading a study group to China in September 2002. Our group made an official visit to the Xiyuan Hospital, a large Traditional Chinese Medicine (TCM) hospital with over 650 beds, treating over 2,000 outpatients each day in various departments.

We spent an afternoon with Dr Xu in the Qigong department after touring the hospital. Dr Xu had a very friendly, approachable, relaxed manner about him as we discussed many ideas regarding Qigong, health and spirituality. He talked about the importance of meditation. When we enter a 'realized state', or the state of nothingness, there is no disease or illness, only nothingness, he explained. The regular practice of meditation will change the energy in our body and mind, helping to cure disease and improve our quality of life. This concept was of great interest to me!

Dr Xu told us he had worked as a barefoot doctor during the Cultural Revolution in the 1970s. He would go out into fields and prescribe different herbs for the workers. When his work proved successful, he was accepted at a university in Wuhan in the Hubei province, where he studied Western Medicine. He worked very hard but suffered from a number of stress-related health conditions. Dr Xu had learnt hard martial Qigong when he was a teenager and started to study the natural healing benefits of Qigong. When he graduated with honors from University, he requested to be posted to the Qigong department at Xiyuan Hospital in Beijing, which was already quite well known. Many highly regarded Masters and doctors were working there, conducting research and using Qigong as a part of their patients' treatment.

From his own research and experience working in this department for over 20 years, Dr Xu has developed a style of Qigong he calls Guigen. 'Guigen' translates to 'returning to the root or source', returning to the primordial energy from which everything emerges. Its six different sections harmonise the different organ meridians in the body. Although our time with Dr Xu was only brief, he kindly taught us the movement 'Stimulating the Water Element' for the kidney and bladder channels. As we left, I told him I would love to return and study more with him, and he gave me an encouraging look and nodded.

When I returned home to Sydney, I had an email from Dr Xu. He enjoys using the internet and has his own website at **www.guigen.cn** He had been looking at my website and congratulated me on the work I've been doing to spread the healing benefits of Qigong in Australia and invited me to study with him at the hospital. We corresponded regularly by email for a few years until I worked out an appropriate time to take a break from my busy teaching schedule and return to Beijing.

I was attending a World Medical Qigong Conference in Beijing in May 2004 and arranged to spend time with Dr Xu on the same trip. He explained that he could either teach me privately at my hotel outside of his working hours at the hospital, or officially at the hospital. However, to be accepted into the hospital for clinical practice, I would need to be a doctor or have some formal qualifications in TCM, and as I don't, he checked with the directors of the hospital. They asked me to submit an account of my training and teaching experience in Qigong. I wrote a brief, 8-page history of my professional background – which you can find on my website – and sent it off to Dr Xu along with my two Qigong DVDs, the Art of Life and Absorbing the Essence. A short time later, he was pleased to inform me that my submission had been accepted.

The World Academic Society of Medical Qigong (WASMQ) had organised the conference I was attending. I had been to one of their previous conferences in Beijing in August 1998 and had become a member. The Chinese Government officially recognises the WASMQ and its importance as an association to help foster the development of Medical Qigong and the international exchange of academic research and training. For the first time, I was presenting a paper which was to be on the work that I had been doing at Drug and Alcohol Rehabilitation Centres in Sydney over the previous 12 years (refer Book 1: The Art of Life). My talk was a great success and I felt quite honored that I could mix with many high level professors, doctors and Qigong Masters.

Because I needed to live in the hospital to receive the certification for clinical practice, Dr Xu had arranged for me to stay in the 'High Official' room there. I had been staying at a luxurious four star hotel during the conference and this arrangement sounded a bit more interesting. But when I arrived at the hospital, Dr Xu told me in his usual joking way, "Sorry, a High Official is staying in your room, so we have organised a nurse's room on the second floor of the inpatient's department for you."

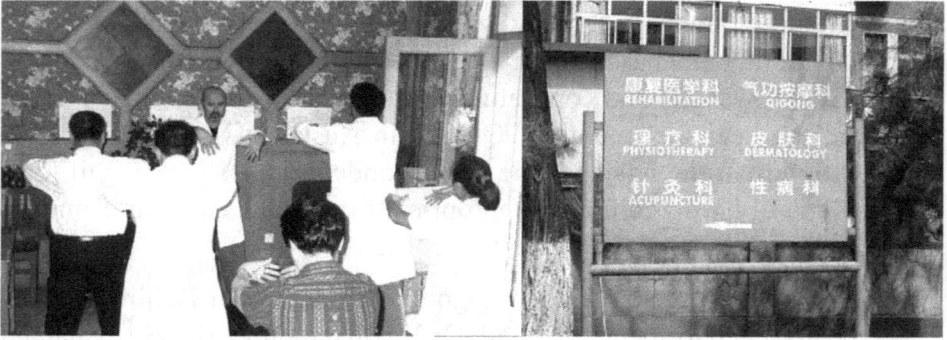

世界卫生组织传统医学合作中心
中 国 中 医 研 究 院 西 苑 医 院
COLLABORATING CENTRE OF TRADITIONAL MEDICINE,
WORLD HEALTH ORGANIZATION OF
XI YUAN HOSPITAL, CHINA ACADEMY OF TRADITIONAL CHINESE MEDICINE

学 习 证 书
CERTIFICATE

编号：200408
NO ：200408

This is to certify that　Simon Blow
From　　Australia
Clinical Practice of　Qigong
In our Hospital
From　　2004.5.18　to　　2004.5.22

兹证明　西蒙·贝洛
从 2004 年 5 月 18 日至 2004 年 5 月 22 日
在我院临床进修 气功

院长盖章：
Seal of the Director:

中 国 中 医 研 究 院
西 苑 医 院

发证日期：2004 年 5 月 22 日
Date of issue: 2004.5.22

I met the directors and other main staff of the hospital and commenced my training as Dr Xu's personal assistant. I would start at 8am at the Qigong clinic and he would teach me the six sections of Guigen Qigong in between patients arriving for treatment. We would break for lunch at 11.30am and recommence at 1pm. From 3pm to 5pm, we held Qigong and meditation practice for patients and other doctors in the department. When word spread that a foreigner was in the Qigong department, a lot of doctors came to meet me, practise their English and discuss what I was studying. Soon, I had a few Qigong students, confirming that the best way to learn is to teach. I could only fit in five days with Dr Xu at the hospital, but we spent valuable time together and shared a common goal and desire to help people improve their quality of life.

On my first morning with Dr Xu, he told me that I was the first Australian Qigong teacher to learn Guigen Qigong and that he wanted me to make a DVD on it so that others could benefit. I produced the DVD 'Qigong - Restoring Natural Harmony' in that same year, 2004, and now this instruction book. I told him I would bring other Qigong teachers and natural therapists to Beijing to learn from him. I organised groups in 2005, 2006 and 2007, with people coming from most states in Australia as well as the UK, Europe and the US. Fifty students received a certificate of Qigong training from the WASMQ and some also became members. Future training tours with Dr Xu are being planned.

I would like to thank Dr Xu for his continued help, support and guidance and also for his friendship and faith in me.

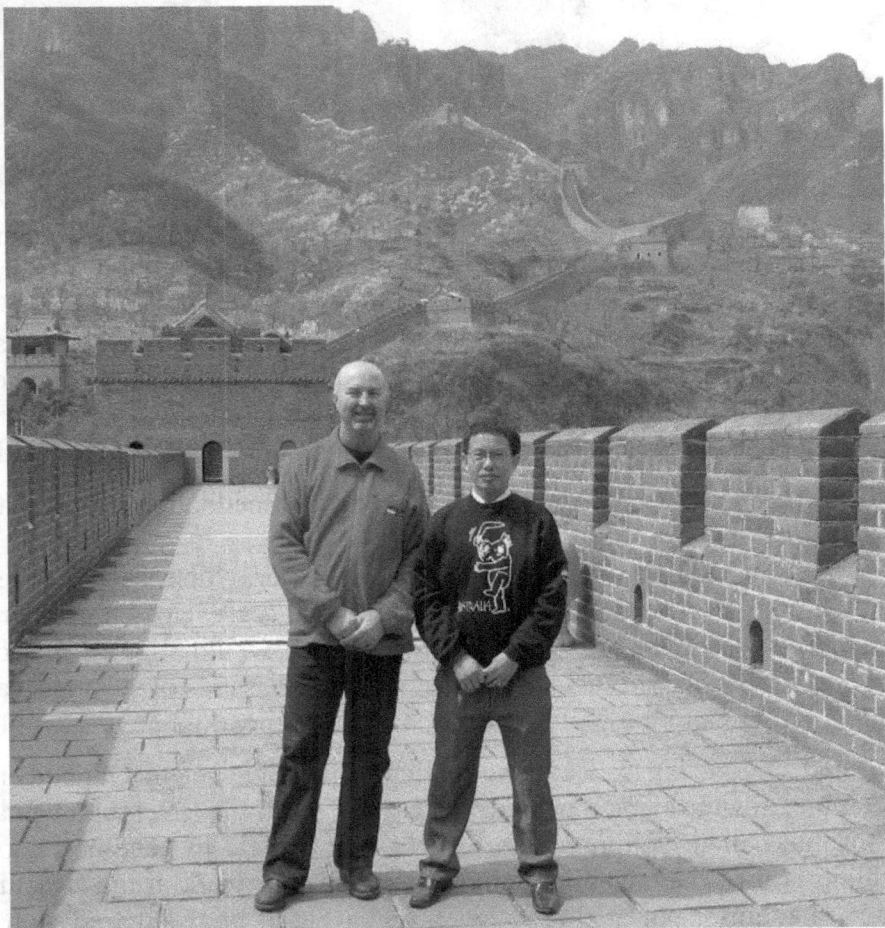

Great Wall of China, Beijing 2007

How can Guigen Qigong treat disease?

The name 'Guigen' translates as 'returning to the source or root'. The six sections of Guigen Qigong help regulate the meridian system, encompassing the ancient Taoist understanding of Restoring Natural Harmony. Combined with Traditional Chinese Medicine practice, it brings harmony to the mind, body and spirit. The dynamic forms and stillness meditation are prescribed to both in- and out-patients at the Xiyuan Hospital as a part of their therapy.

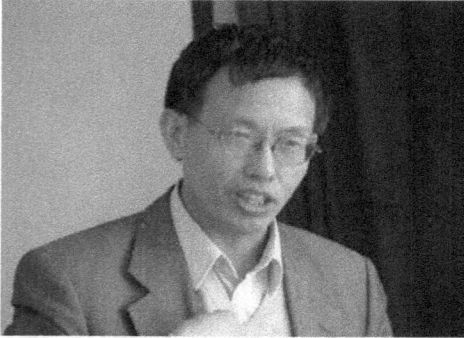

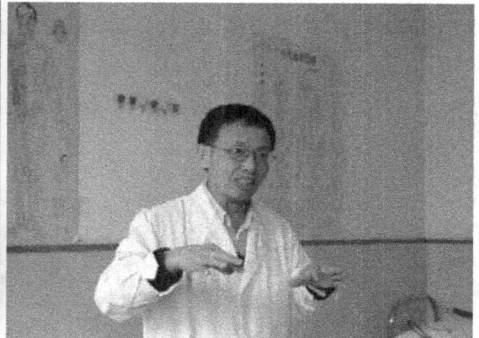

According to Dr Xu, there are three different types of medicine: structural, functional and energetic. We seek treatment for various conditions relating to these types. If we have a fractured arm, we need the structure to be set and to allow the natural healing process to take place. Similarly, if we have a problem with our internal organs, we need herbs or other medications to adjust their function. Qigong works on the Qi or energy level, with the building blocks that help maintain the structure and function of the body.

When asked to describe how Guigen Qigong and meditation treat disease, Dr Xu answers:

"In different medical systems, the meaning of the term 'disease' is different. But Qigong has an effect on most chronic diseases to some degree. According to conventional medical theory, this would suggest that one Qigong system should include not just six but thousands of sections, each addressing one of many different 'diseases', which would be impossible.

"Instead, Qigong is a truly holistic healing knowledge system. Our body has a complex diagnostic and healing system that I call the 'internal hospital', a hospital called Nothingness, all inclusive. Critical to genuine Qigong healing is the understanding that Qigong does not work at the structural level (anatomy), but at the Qi level, or Qi based knowledge system or framework, even beyond the Qi dimension. Your question was about what kinds of diseases can be treated by Qigong, or which section applies to which disease.

"Disease is a term based on sensational knowing, but to practise Qigong effectively, the first step is to put aside all sensations. For example, for a doctor to give someone a diagnosis of gastric ulcer, he first needs to know the patient's symptoms, such as "pain in upper abdomen" or "tender in the local area" and then carry out an examination. These initial procedures, based on sensation, give the doctor clues about the cause of the problem – gastritis, gastric ulcer or tumour, for example. Next, he may prescribe an investigation by gastroscope, a visual examination perhaps indicating some structural abnormality. He may perform a biopsy under the microscope – another visual technique – to determine whether an ulcer or inflammation is benign or malignant.

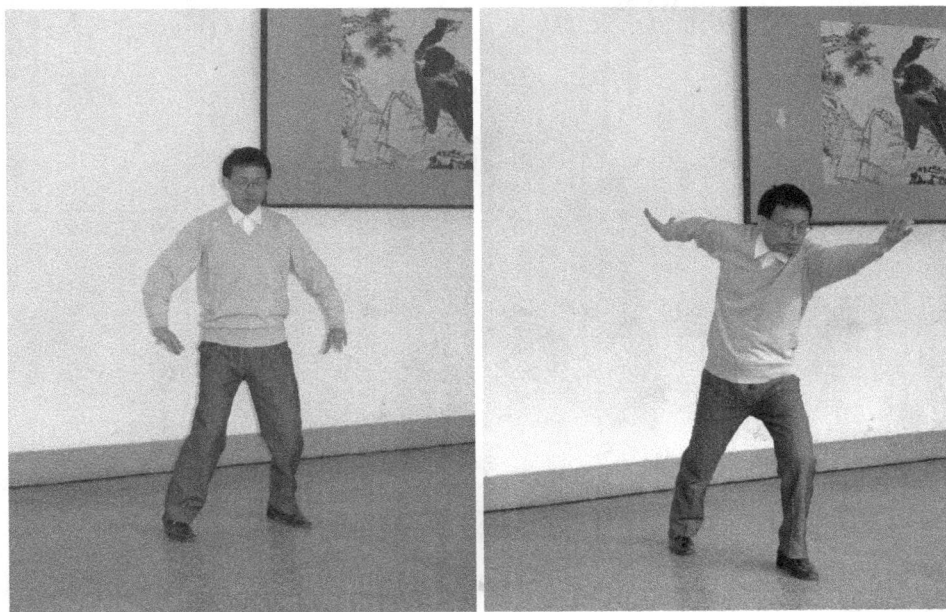

Dr Xu demonstrating Guigen Qigong, Section 1 and Section 6.

"TCM and Qigong practitioners, however, work on Qi, not on diseases. They treat the Qi stagnations and make them flow smoothly and easily. When the Qi system is genuinely fixed or repaired, the problems in the structural dimension (diseases) will be healed very quickly. This is why we emphasise, "Nothingness is the best prescription." If your internal diagnostic system scans your Qi system and finds nothing, it means that there is no stagnation in your Qi dimension, and your Qi-body is normal.

The Qi-body is the root or source of the structure-body. Qigong cures the 'diseases' in the body through repairing Qi.

"Although I don't list diseases such as cancers (of the breast, prostate, uterus, stomach, intestines), chronic inflammations (mostly caused by viruses, bacteria, physical and chemical factors, autoimmune factors), emotional and mental problems, metabolic diseases (overweight, diabetes, coronary heart disease and rest enosis) or insomnia, most chronic diseases are included. To obtain a better result, the following conditions should be met. First, the patient should be very willing and open to resolving their problems through Qigong practice. Second, the patient must have the energy and ability for daily practice. These two are the basic requirements for Qigong self-healing. The first is more important than the second. If the patient's practice abides by the general principles of Qigong, good results will appear naturally."

Thank you
Yours,
Dr Xu
www.guigen.cn

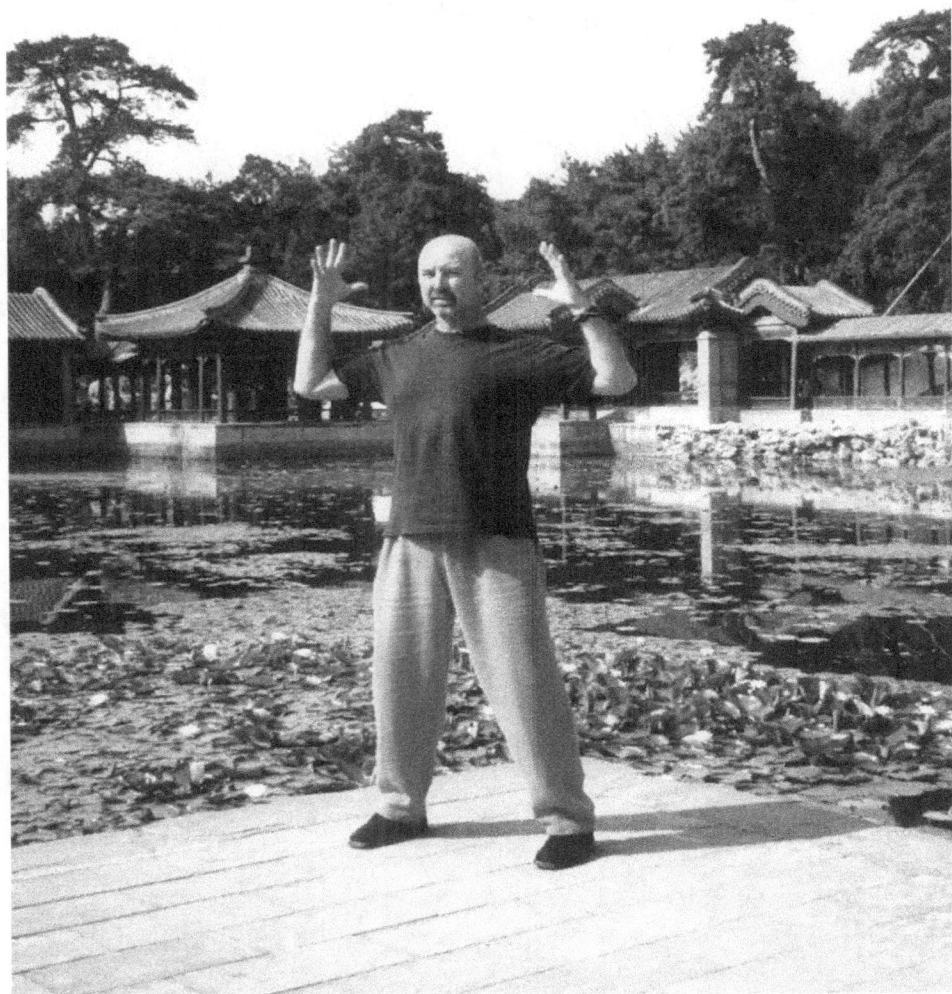

Summer Palace, Beijing 2004

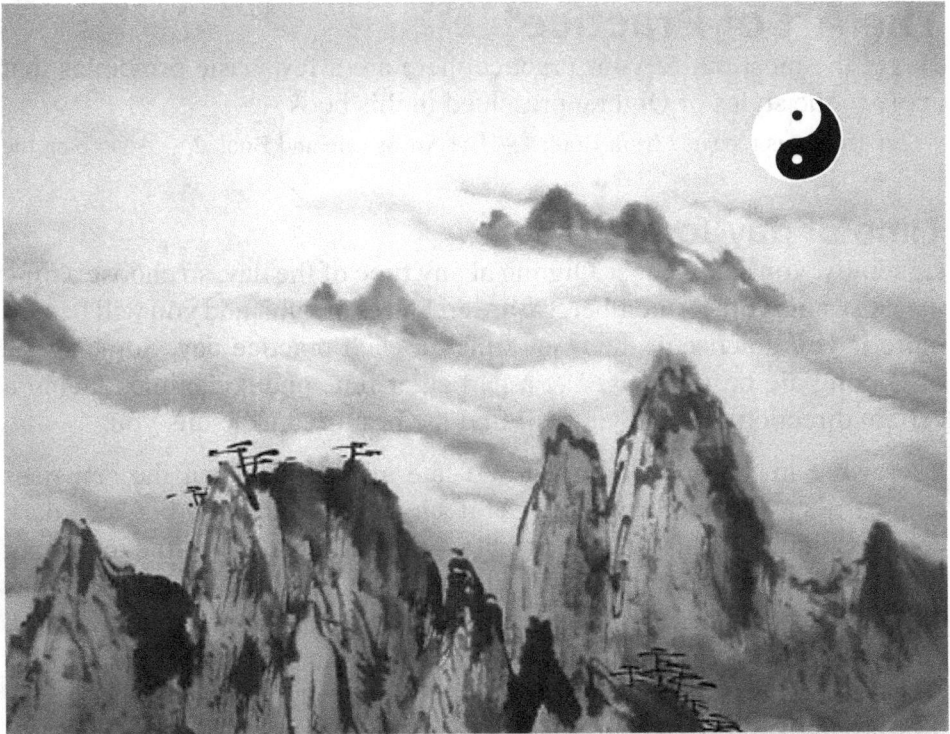

Chapter 3

The Art of Practice

Restoring Natural Harmony

The Art of Practice*

To get the most out of your practice there are a few basic principles that apply to the styles of Qigong presented in this book.

* This section is repeated from Book 1 – The Art of Life and Book 2 – Absorbing the Essence

Time of day to practise

Generally, you can practise Qigong at any time of the day, so choose a time that best suits you. Remember, we are creatures of habit and you will benefit more if you practise at the same time on each practice day. Some styles of Qigong are best practised at a particular time and sometimes facing a certain direction. In time you will find the best time that suits you.

Exercising in the early morning and late afternoon, when the sun rises and sets, is a very powerful time as it's a natural transition between dark coolness of night (Yin) and the bright warmth of day (Yang). It's important not to look directly into the sun in the early morning or late afternoon as this can cause damage to your eyes. The setting of the sun and transition between Yang and Yin is a time when nature has a great influence on your body. You might notice that birds are very active at this time of the day, as they are in the morning.

I am often asked by new students if it's best to practise with the eyes open or closed, and what does one look at when practising. It may be easier to concentrate when the eyes are closed as we are not distracted by things around us, but the general rule with Qigong is to have the eyes open when moving, looking to the distance but not really looking. Your awareness is on the external (Yang) when the eyes are open and you can absorb the energy or Qi from the environment and universe. It's OK to momentarily close the eyes but it's important to keep them open – not too wide, and relaxed. When practising Qigong meditation or Neigong the eyes are closed as your awareness is now on the internal (Yin).

As a rule, you should not exercise on a full or empty stomach. Instead of eating breakfast, consume liquids as they stimulate stomach-intestine movement which acts as an internal massage. Warm or room temperature water is the best with a slice of lemon. Cold water from the fridge interferes with Qi circulation.

Qigong exercise in the evenings is a way to free your mind and body from the burdens of a busy day and a way of processing the events of the day and letting things go, physically and emotionally. Students often comment on how they get their best night's sleep after attending class. You will then be able to sleep more quietly and recover more fully because the body begins its recovery during Qigong and this continues during sleep.

"When I practise my Qigong in the evening, I sleep much better. Therefore I have more energy the next day." Cherel Waters

We are all a bit different. I wouldn't advise that you practise immediately before going to sleep as it stimulates your energy and may disrupt your sleep. But a few students have told me that when they haven't been able to sleep they get up and practise which calms their mind and body. They then have a restful sleep.

Eating and drinking

For Qigong exercise you need a clear head. Beverages such as alcohol, tea and coffee affect concentration and body functions and if you are not calm and relaxed you will not feel the full benefits of Qigong exercise. It's best to avoid drinking cold fluids during or immediately after practice as this interferes with Qi circulation.

When I was training with Master Ho we began early in the morning at 6.30am and he would take my pulse before and after practice. A few times he became very concerned as my heart rate and organ functions were erratic. He watched me very closely, my movements were slow and smooth and my breath deep and even. After a lot of questions I told him I had a strong espresso coffee half an hour before we started. I have now changed my morning routine and only have warm water or green tea.

Avoid exercising on either an empty stomach or after a full meal. Being distracted by hunger will not help your mental focus so if you are hungry, have something light to eat or something to drink. A full stomach interferes with Qi circulation. The Qi is diverted into the digestive system as stomach juices increase and stomach-intestinal movements occur, leaving very little Qi to circulate elsewhere.

When not to exercise

When we exercise we absorb the good influences from nature and the macrocosm. Similarly, we absorb the influences from turbulent weather conditions. Therefore, it is not good to practise Qigong during bad weather, heavy fog, extreme heat, before or during a thunderstorm, on excessively windy days, or during lunar or solar eclipses. Exercise can begin again when nature is balanced.

Menstruation and pregnancy

Basic Qigong is good to practise during menstruation and pregnancy as it will improve the circulation of Qi, blood and other body fluids.

Women who are menstruating should pay attention to the effects of Qigong exercise. If the exercise produces a negative effect, stop immediately and continue when feeling better.

Special care is also required during pregnancy. Each woman's pregnancy is different, and it is recommended that the expectant mother consult her primary care provider as well as a qualified and experienced Qigong teacher.

"I attended Simon's week-long retreat during my pregnancy and experienced a great release of muscle tension particularly in my arms and shoulders. I also found the meditation that followed the Qigong practice easy to do even though I had never meditated before. It was a very pleasurable experience." Jessica Henley

Where to practise

Qigong can be practised anywhere but some places are better than others. It's best to be undisturbed during Qigong practice to help maintain a concentrated mind. The best places are in nature in the open air where the Heaven (Yang) and Earth (Yin) Qi are most abundant such as in the mountains, beside a waterfall or by the ocean. Near a waterfall or by the ocean is excellent because moving water generates lots of Qi.

If you are practising indoors, try to find a quiet and peaceful space away from draughts, with natural light and fresh air. Avoid excessive noise, TV sets and computers and turn off your mobile phone or set it to silent.

The proximity of some plants should also be avoided. The Oleander plant for example, is known to be poisonous and has a very tense Qi. As you practise you will learn which plants feel relaxing and harmonious. Lovely flowers and large old trees are ideal.

What to wear

There are no rules regarding clothing but since relaxation is important in Qigong try to wear loose comfortable clothing, ideally made of natural fibres such as cotton or silk.

If you are limited in what you can wear, for example if you are at work, loosen your collar and tie, your belt/waistband and remove uncomfortable or high heel shoes. It's important that you wear flat soled shoes or even bare feet are OK. I always wear soft sports shoes as I damaged my feet and ankles a long time ago and I find wearing shoes gives me a bit more support. It's a personal preference. There are many light, soft shoes around today.

Whatever clothing you choose to wear it should not be tight around the waist because the Qi needs to flow easily. Preferably, remove watches and bracelets as they restrict the flow of Qi through the wrist.

If it is chilly, dress appropriately. Feeling cold during a Qigong session can decrease the effectiveness of the exercises particularly if your hands, belly and back are cold. Chilling your kidneys severely restricts your Qi circulation. I often start my practice on colder mornings with gloves, hat and a warm jacket and I can always take them off.

How long to practise

The benefits that are gained from Qigong are proportional to the amount of practice. For beginners, an exercise period of 15 to 30 minutes daily is recommended in order to relax the body and mind and feel the Qi. It is only when the body's carriage is regulated according to Qigong principles that the Qi will flow easily and the benefits of Qigong realised. If you can achieve 30 minutes twice a day, you will notice a marked increase in vitality and peace within a few weeks. If you have major health issues and can manage a couple of hours per day you will soon see a radical improvement in your health and wellbeing. Regardless of your state of health when you begin, any amount of regular practice will improve how you feel.

"I have practised Qigong every day for sixteen years. It helps bring me right into the present moment with a feeling of immense serenity. Each year my health has improved and whenever I experience a set-back, gentle Qigong is always there to help me." Joan Downey

"Over the last few years I have been practising five to six times per week. I am in my 80th year and have gone from wearing a hinged metal knee brace to wearing no brace at all. My knee still creaks but is no longer painful and range of movement is barely restricted." Shirley Chittick

How long does the effect of Qigong exercise last?

Qigong works because the Qi is brought into order and the mind, body and spirit are in harmony. This harmony can be disturbed by arguing, getting excited or annoyed, engaging in strenuous physical activity, eating excessively, and even going to the toilet. If possible, use the toilet beforehand rather than after Qigong exercise because urination and defecation bring the Qi into definite motion.

I often tell my students after a Qigong class that if they have driven a car to get to the class try not to play the radio when they leave because all the senses have been enhanced and body functions are in harmony. In the quietness and stillness you may get good ideas, solve some problems, or if you are with friends you might have some amazing conversations. Look at the beauty of the sky, trees, the divine in all living things. I love to look at clouds. It's a creative time, so use it wisely and the Qi will be with you longer. The more you cultivate your Qi the more in harmony with the universe you will be, improving all aspects of your life.

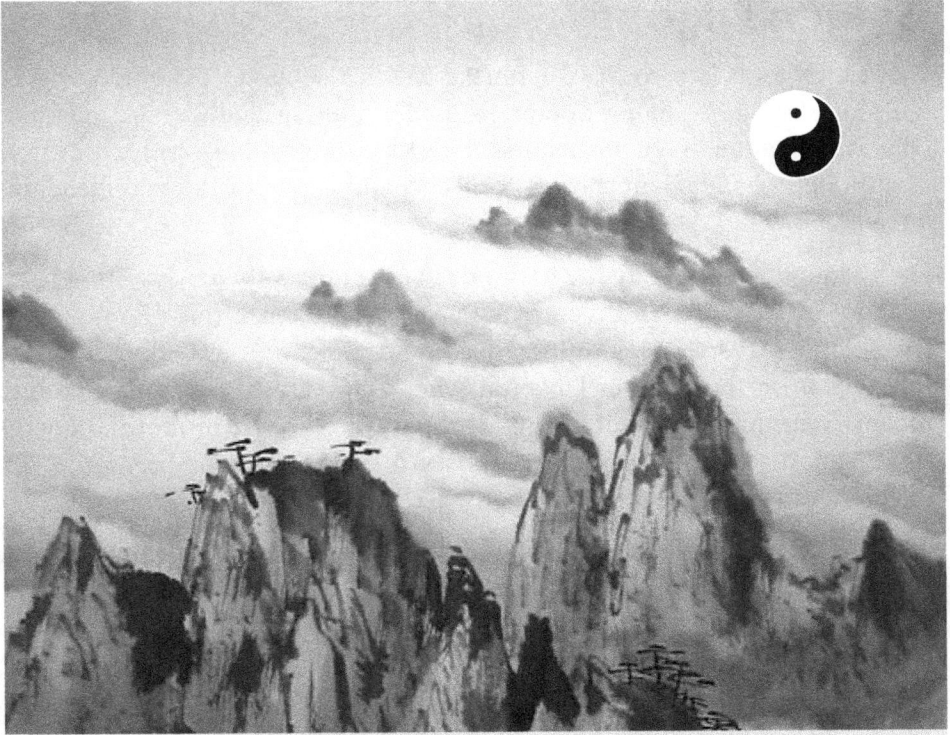

Chapter 4

Guigen Qigong

歸根氣功

Restoring Natural Harmony

Guigen Qigong

Guigen Qigong is a form of Chinese Medical Qigong developed by Dr Xu Hongtao, a specialist doctor from the Qigong and Tuina (massage) Department at the Xiyuan Hospital. The Xiyuan Hospital was built in 1949 as a model for the advancement for TCM and is one of the main teaching hospitals in China.

Dr Xu taught Guigen Qigong methods to me personally in May 2004 at his hospital in Beijing and gave me authorisation to teach this Qigong form. I was granted World Health Organisation certification in Qigong Clinical Practice from the Xiyuan Hospital where Dr Xu has his clinic. Guigen means returning to the root or source, returning to the primordial energy from which everything emerges. Its six different sections harmonise the different organ meridians in the body, Restoring Natural Harmony.

Movement: The posture should be upright and relaxed and the movements carried out at a smooth, even pace without speeding up or slowing down, remembering that we are only guiding the Qi, allowing it to restore natural harmony.

Breathing: The breath should also be smooth and even, in and out through the nose in coordination with the movement. As a general rule, when the hands come closer to the body, breathe in and allow the Qi to envelope the organ that you are working on. When breathing out, the hands come away from the body, dispersing the stale Qi. In time and with regular practice, don't concentrate on the breath too much but allow the movement and the breath to coordinate naturally.

Mind: Once you have gained confidence in the movements and the breath is flowing smoothly, mental concentration is an important element of practising Guigen Qigong. A controlled, relaxed focus is better than concentrating too much. As Dr Xu advises, the Qi knows where to go.

Dan Tian: This translates to 'the field where the elixir or energy grows'. It is one of the major energy centres of the body and is situated just below the navel. It's like a storehouse or reservoir where the cultivated Qi energy is stored for later use. After practising Guigen Qigong we place our hands in this area, one hand on top of the other, with Loa Gong points (in palm of hands) connected, then allowing your breath, mind and energy to settle. See diagram in the chapter Meditation Points, at the back of this book.

Basic principles

Qi is a flowing energy and is often compared to water. When water flows through a river system, the environment, plants and animals gain nourishment from this fresh energy supply and will be in good health. When this flow of water becomes blocked or stagnates, the environment around it suffers. I don't think there is good and bad energy – it's all just energy. Similarly, after rain, the stagnant water flows again through the network of channels, streams and along the major rivers giving life again to the environment.

Our own body is a micro representation of our environment and works similarly to the river system. With the correct approach, we can cultivate and transform the stagnant energy in our body into fresh sustaining energy. This flow of Qi in our body is directly related to our posture and body movements, breath and mental condition. When the mind, body and breath are in harmony, our Qi will also be in harmony. It will flow naturally through the energy channels or meridians of the body and with loving kindness, we as conscious beings are able to let our energy or Qi merge with the energy of the universe.

When we practise Qigong, it's important not to try too hard. Take your time, allowing the movements and the breath to develop. Firstly, we concentrate on the body posture, either standing or sitting, keeping the spine upright and letting the muscles and flesh relax around the skeleton. The movements of Qigong help clear the energy blockages in our body. Also known as guiding Qi, your movements will become slow, soft and smooth with regular practice. Then we can concentrate on the breath.

There are a number of different breathing patterns for different styles of Qigong. For the styles presented here, we breathe in and out through the nose to the abdominal area, slowly, deeply and deliberately. When we breathe in, the abdomen gently expands and when breathing out, it gently contracts. This is known as natural breathing. In time, the breath will naturally coordinate with the movements, helping the mind focus and allowing a fusion between mind, body and breath.

The practice of Qigong should become a pleasurable experience and when you are practising correctly, a gentle, natural smile will permeate throughout the whole body, from the heart through every cell. As Qigong Grand Master Jack Lim often told me, you can tell if a student has understood a lesson, not by their performance of the movements, but by the smile at the end of the class.

These basic principles apply to all styles of Qigong:

1. Regulating the posture and movement
2. Regulating the breath
3. Regulating the mind

When the mind, body and breath are in harmony, our Qi will also be in harmony.

Basic stance

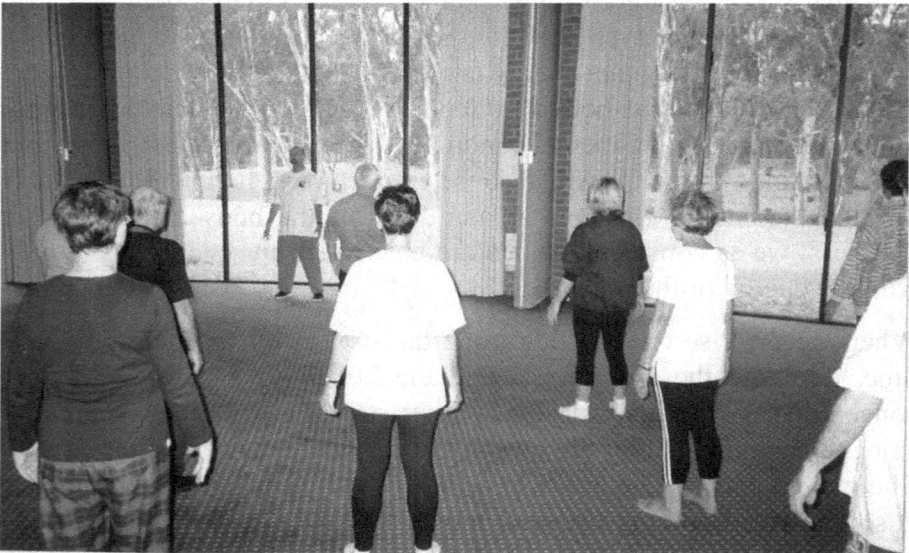

There are many ways to prepare for Qigong practice but the basic stance is the foundation of most styles of Qigong. Stand with feet parallel, shoulder-width apart, as if standing on train tracks. Knees are slightly off lock. Let your weight sink into your legs, feet and into the ground. Keep the coccyx or tail bone slightly tucked in, chest relaxed, and the back straight. Hold your arms away from the body, fingers open and relaxed pointing to the earth, palms facing the body.

With the chin slightly tucked in and the top of the head (Bai Hui point) reaching to the sky as if a silken cord attached to it is lifting the whole body, light the Hui Yin by gently squeezing the pelvic floor. Relax your eyes and face and look out into the distance. Keeping your jaw relaxed, place the tip of your tongue on the top palate of your mouth, just behind the front teeth. Breathe in and out through the nose. When breathing in, let the abdomen push out slightly and as the breath comes out, let the abdomen contract. Just relax, letting the whole body breathe.

With the eyes closed, allow the breath to become smooth and even, and let your mind rest. After a few breaths, concentrate on the out-breath, relaxing from the top of the head to the soles of the feet. Just relax down through the body on the out-breath. After a few more breaths, let the knees and hips sink a bit closer to the ground and feel the pressure go into the feet. Like a tree, follow the roots from the soles of your feet deeply into the ground. As you let the breath out, relax down through the body into the ground, letting the stress and tension of the body dissolve into the earth.

After another few breaths, with your awareness, push up the spine one vertebra at a time, checking that the chin tucks in and letting the head pull away from the body. We seem to stand taller as the top of the head reaches up and touches the sky. Stay in this posture for a few breaths, feeling the peace. With your eyes gradually opening, look out into the distance.

Qigong warm-up

The warm-up exercises that I have developed for most of the Qigong practices that I teach are not only a way of preparing the mind and body for the Qigong movements that follow, they are also very good exercise. Physically, when we rotate and loosen the joints we exercise the ligaments and tendons, as well as the membranes that secrete synovial fluid to lubricate the joints. Energetically, we clear stagnant energy (Qi) that can accumulate around the joints.

These warm-up exercises are not included on this DVD, therefore they are not included in this book. However, if you would like to see or read about the warm-up exercises they are available in my first two book/DVD sets – 'Book 1: The Art of Life' and 'Book 2: Absorbing the Essence'

Commencement and closing movement

This energetic opening and closing movement is practised at the beginning and end of each section of Guigen Qigong. It is important to relax the whole body and let the mental energy, the excessive Yang Qi, descend, clearing the mind. This movement gathers and brings the Heaven Qi (Yang) down to the top of the head (Bai Hui point) like an energy shower, permeating every cell of the body.

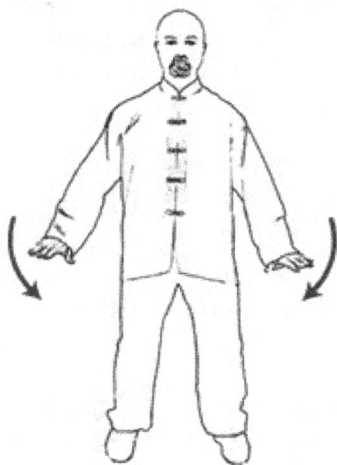

A

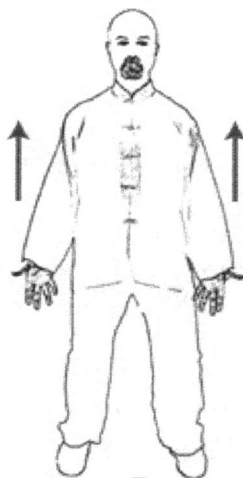

B

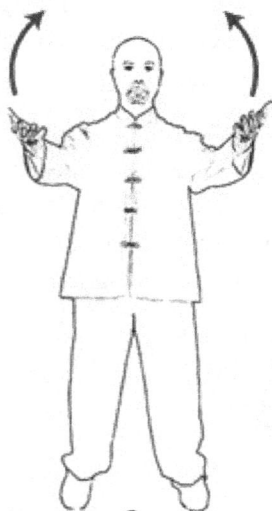

C

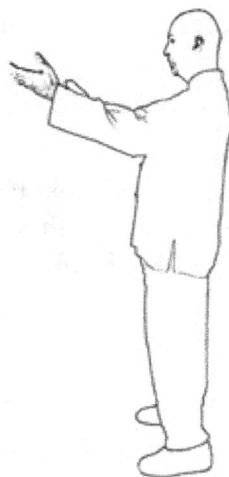

D

A, B, Scoop hands down, gathering earth Qi (Yin), then up in
C, D front of body up high overhead.

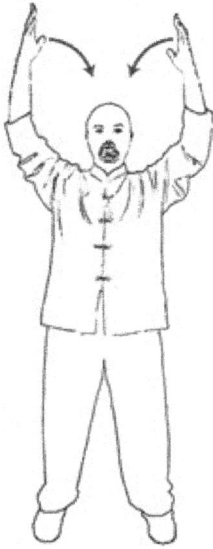 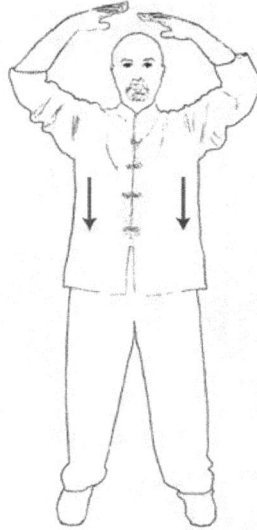 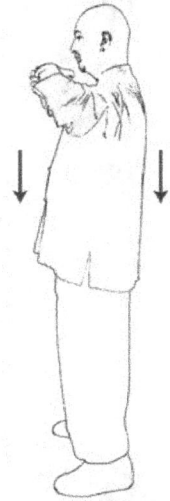

| E | F | G |

E, F, Breathing in, gather and bring the Heaven Qi (Yang) down to the
G top of the head (Bai Hui point), breathing out, and bring hands down
in front of the body, palms facing down.

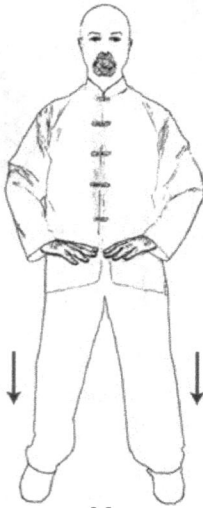

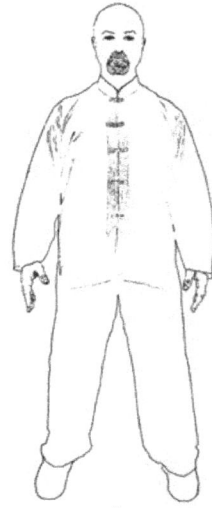

H   **I**

H, I Separate the hands as they reach the navel (Dan Tian), with fingers
pointing to the ground. Allow the Heaven Qi to permeate the whole
body both inside and out like an energy shower, cleansing and healing
the whole body, to the soles of the feet (Yong Chuan, Gushing Spring
point) and into the earth.

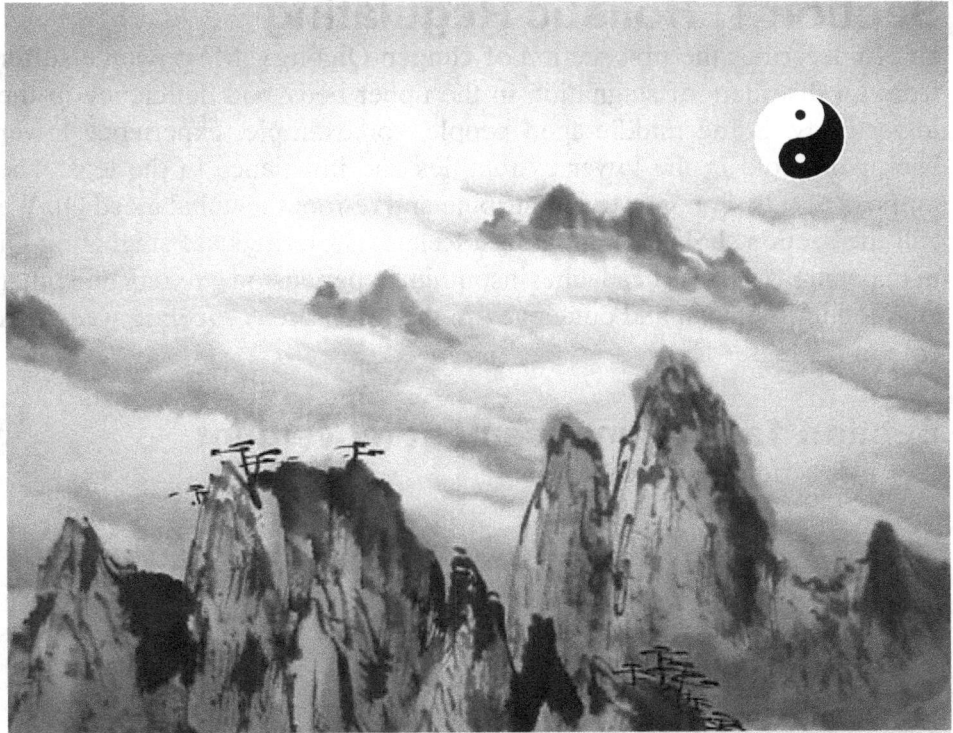

Chapter 5

Section 1: Holistic Regulating

Restoring Natural Harmony

Section 1: Holistic Regulating

Dr Xu describes the first section of Guigen Qigong: "Most people suffer from Qi disorders of stagnation in the upper body and deficiency in the lower body. Some middle-aged people, for example, experience lower back pain, cold in the lower extremities and imbalance in the legs. The purpose of this section is to redistribute and re-root the unbalanced Qi. We call the section 'holistic regulating'. Related sufferings are stagnating Qi in upper areas such as headache, insomnia, hypertension, anxiety and other emotional problems, and deficiency in the lower areas - feeling weak and cold in the legs."

Section 1a: Commencement movement

(See instructions page 30)

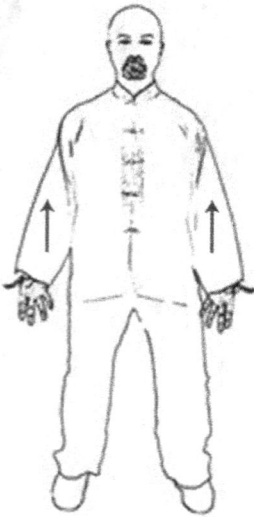

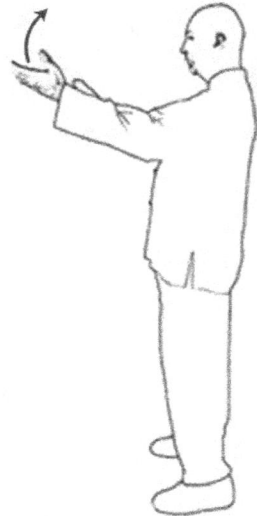

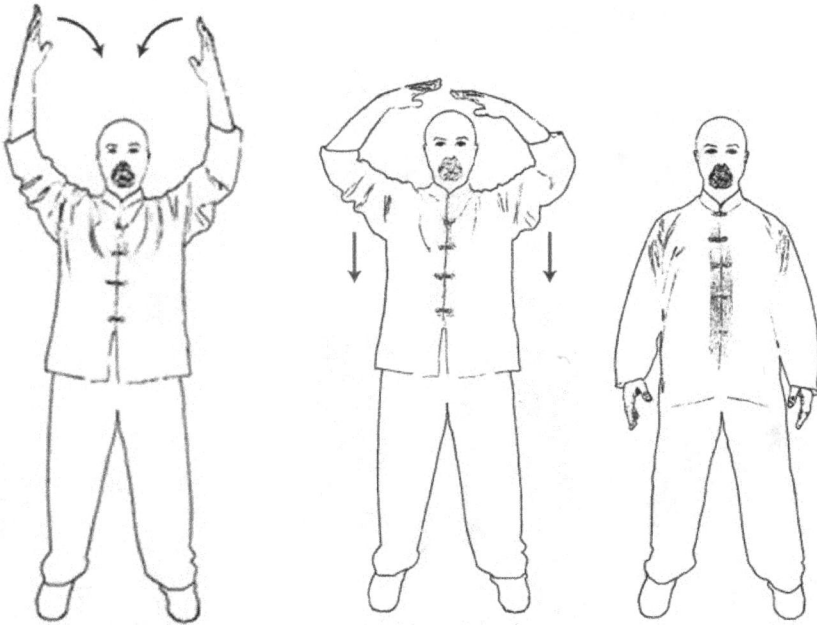

Section 1b: Holistic regulating

Please note that the images are mirrored to the reader; just follow in the same direction.

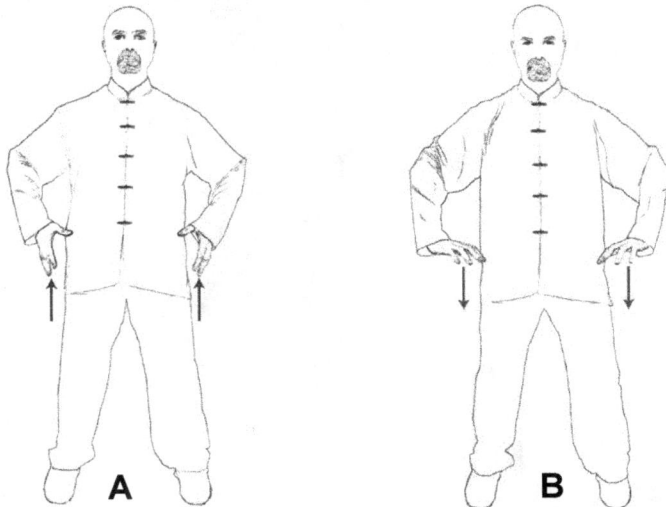

A, B   With hands relaxed at your sides, raise the arms, fingers pointing down and towards the body. Push hands down as if holding a ball floating in water at waist height. Make sure the thumb and fingers are separated (tiger's mouth open). At the same time, lower the legs in coordination with your arms.

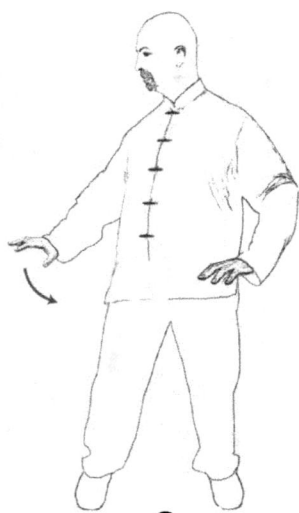

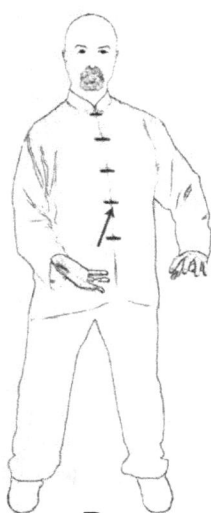

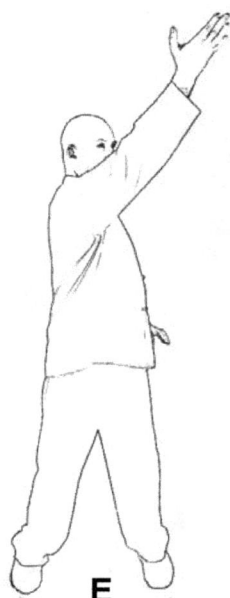

C　　　　　**D**　　　　　**E**

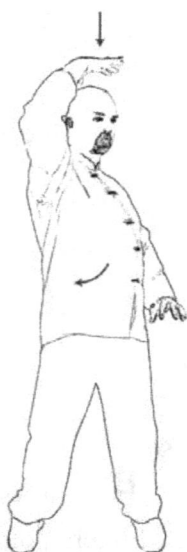

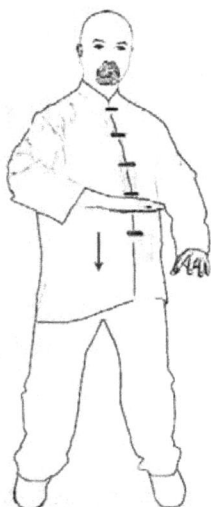

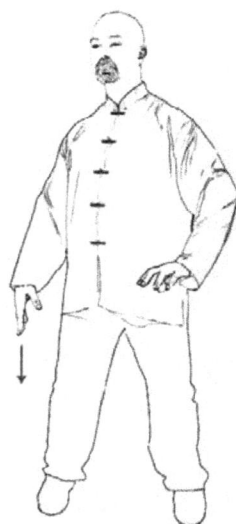

F　　　　　**G**　　　　　**H**

C, D,   Scoop the left hand across your body up high overhead, turning
E   from the waist 90° to the right, eyes following the hand.

F, G   Turn the palm to the top of your head (Bai Hui) and guide the Qi
down as the hand moves down in front of the body, turning back
from the waist.

H   When the left hand is in front of the Dan Tian, let the fingers point
down, allowing stale Qi to dissolve into the earth.

Section 1c

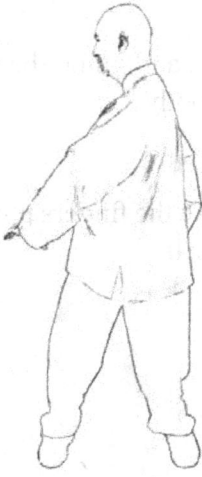

FRONT VIEW

A

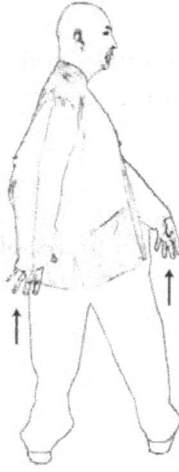

BACK VIEW

A

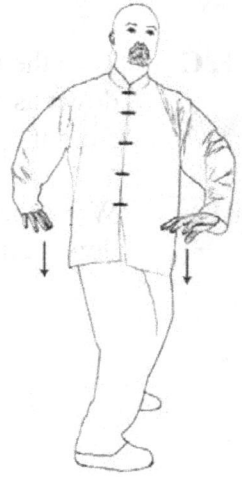

SIDE VIEW

A

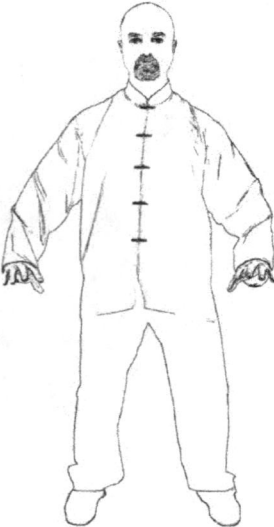

B

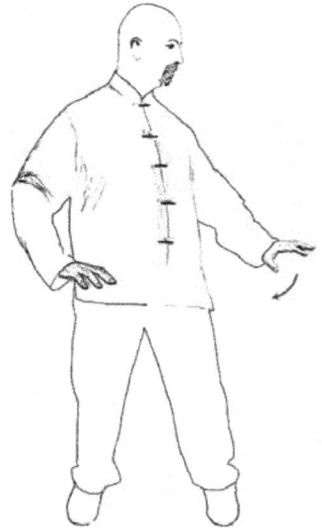

C

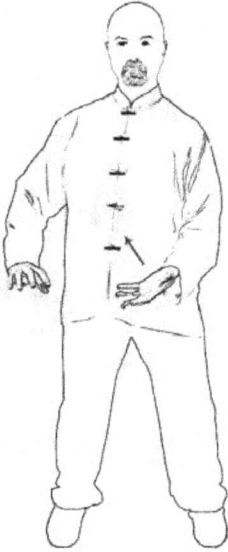

D

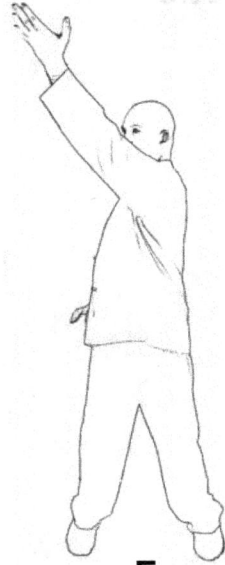

E

A With the right hand still holding floating ball, continue turning left, turning from the waist, until the shoulders are at 90° to the feet and the left hand is over right heel, the right hand is over left toe. Relax hands. With fingers pointing to ground, raise the hands and then push down, as if gently holding down floating balls.

B Relax the right hand, extend fingers with palm facing down, turning from the waist to your right, palm soft as if patting a cat, left hand still holding the floating ball.

C, D, When your right hand reaches the right hip, scoop up and turn
E. from the waist 90° to the left, up high overhead, eyes following the hand.

Section 1d

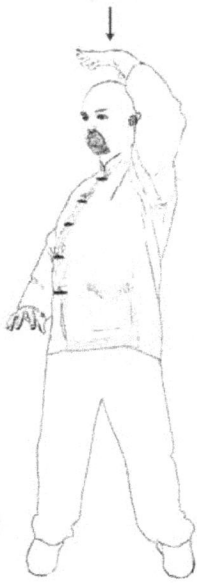

A

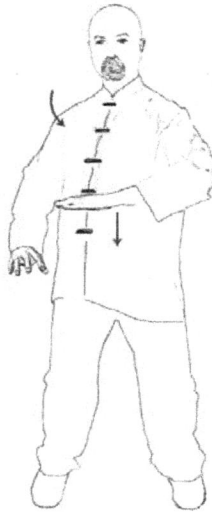

B

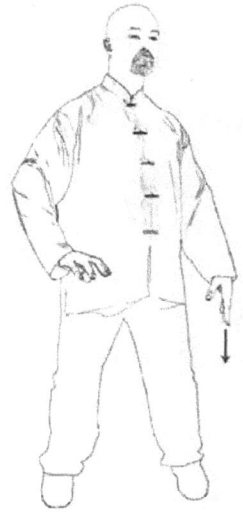

C

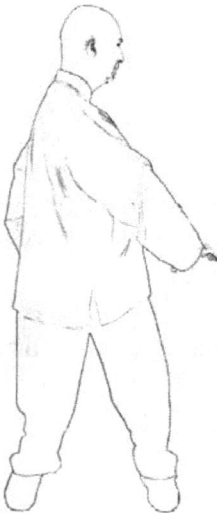

D

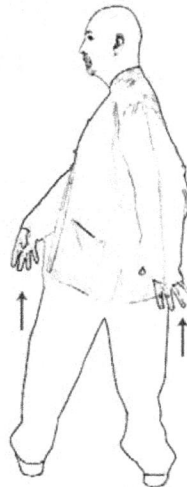

BACK VIEW

E

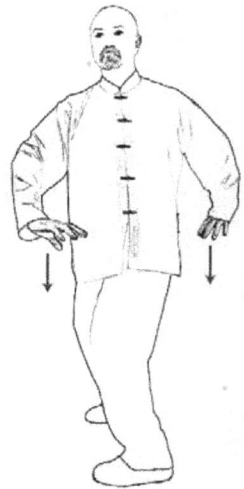

SIDE VIEW

F

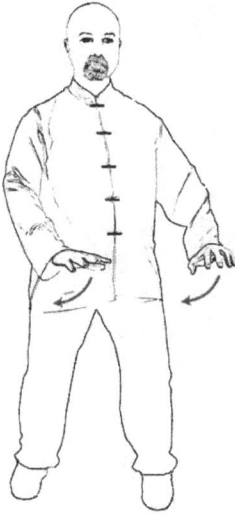

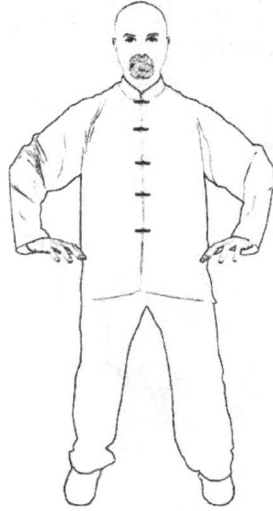

G

H

A, B   Turn palm to top of head (Bai Hui) and guide Qi down as hand moves down in front of body, turning from waist.

C   When the right hand is in front of the Dan Tian, let the fingers point down, allowing stale Qi to dissolve into the earth.

D   With the left hand still holding the ball, continue turning from the waist now to the right until your right hand is over the left heel and the left hand is over the right toe. Relax your hands, fingers pointing to the ground.

E, F   Now raise the hands, and then push down as if gently holding down floating balls.

G, H   Turn to the front from the waist with both hands holding down floating balls.

Finish with closing movement

(See instructions page 30)

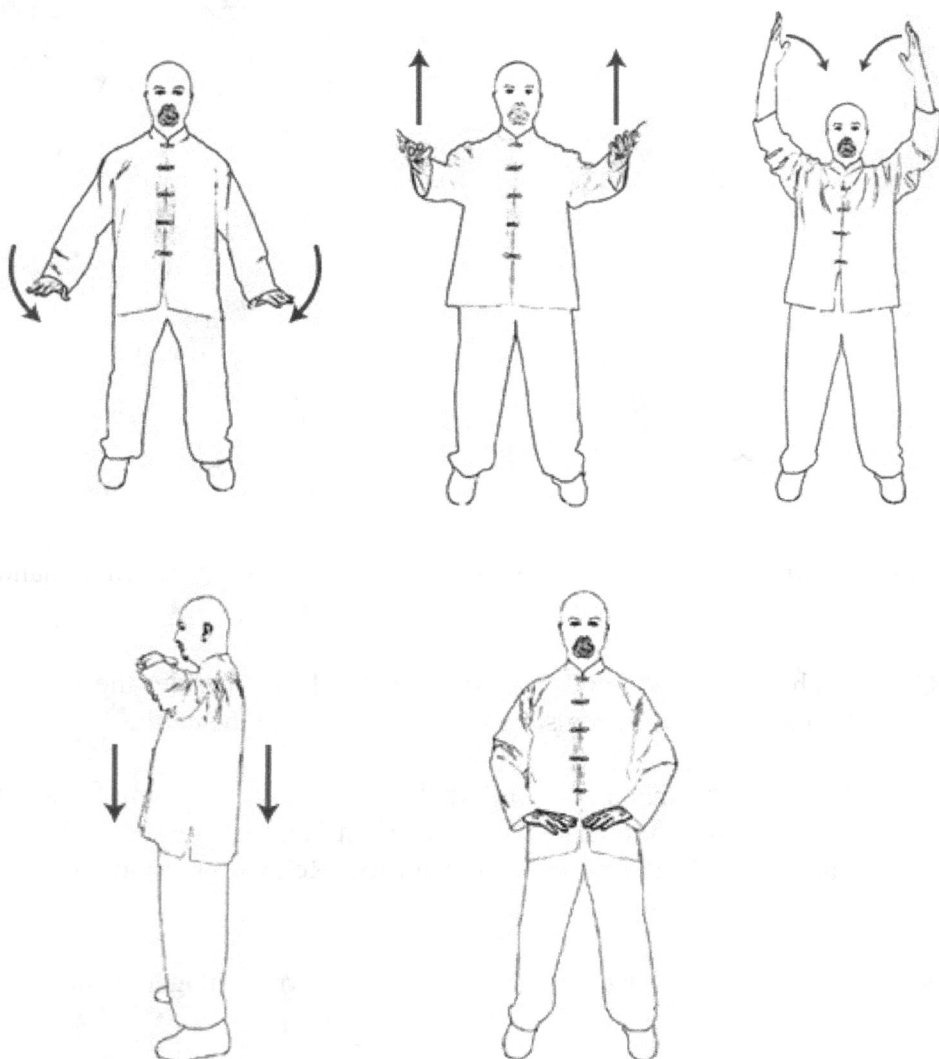

Repeat section No. 1 again to the other side, starting with the right hand scooping to the left then up high overhead.

While practising 'Holding Floating Balls', draw the energy (Qi) of the earth to the fingers when raising the hands and bring the Qi into the hands when holding down the floating balls. Remember to keep all the joints relaxed as if holding a ball or balloon floating in water.

Chapter 6

Section 2: The Earth Element

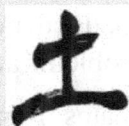

土

Restoring Natural Harmony

Section 2: The Earth Element relates to the spleen (Yin) and stomach (Yang).

The Indian late summer and the climate of humidity correspond to the Earth Element, as does the colour golden yellow. Deep thinking and worry relate to the spleen and anxiety relates to the pancreas.

The spleen is located on the left side of the abdominal area and is the main organ of the digestive system in TCM. The functions of the pancreas and the mouth also relate to the spleen which, according to TCM, is where food and fluids enter the body. The stomach digests the food, sending solids and fluids down, while the essence of these nutrients is sent up to the spleen. The spleen transforms this essence and distributes it to the rest of the body.

Unlike wood, the earth cannot reach toward the sky to actively gather up the Qi. The earth's nature is rather to keep still, to receive, absorb and contain the Qi, and to nourish life. When people have weak Earth Qi, they can worry excessively and are prone to pensiveness. They may overwork, especially in studying or other intellectual work. Worry and anxious thinking has a very negative effect on Earth Qi. The more Qi we expend through worry and useless mental activity, the less we have available to move forward on our life path. Meditation can quieten the mind's random chatter and engaging in Qigong can quieten it further as psychic Qi is moved back into the vital cycles of life.

Dr Xu describes the benefits of section 2: "It is designed to treat the problems of the mouth, stomach, duodenum, spleen (the term spleen is the term of TCM, small intestine problems are included.)"

The Spleen channel (Yin) originates from the outside of the big toe, to the ankle, and rises up the inside of the leg to the hip, through the abdomen to the chest. The Stomach channel (Yang) originates from beneath the eye, down to the corner of the mouth, around the jaw, and descends down the neck to the nipple, down the centre of the body to the pubic bone. From the hip, it continues down the front of the leg, passing the knee to the middle of the front of the ankle and finishing on the outside of the second toe.

The Spleen Channel

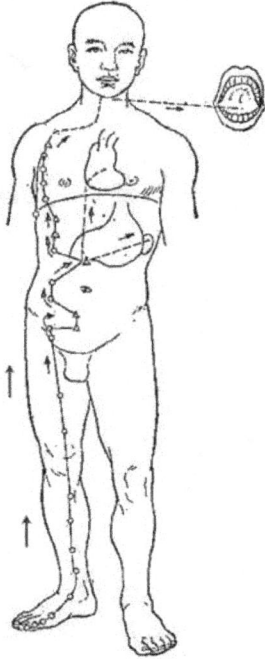

The Stomach Channel

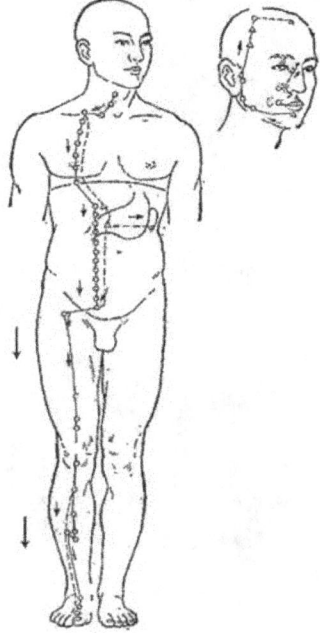

Section 2a: Commencement movement

(See instructions page 30)

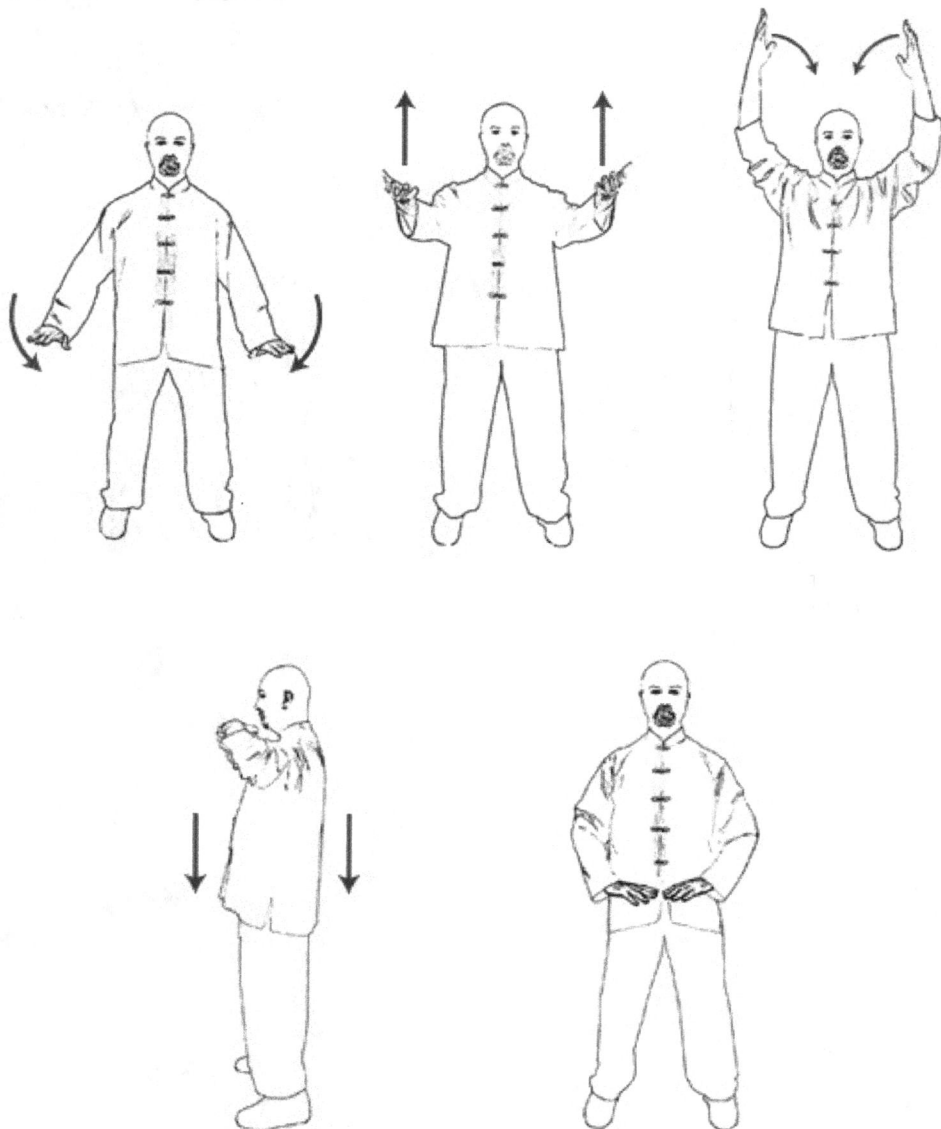

Section 2b: Spleen and stomach movement

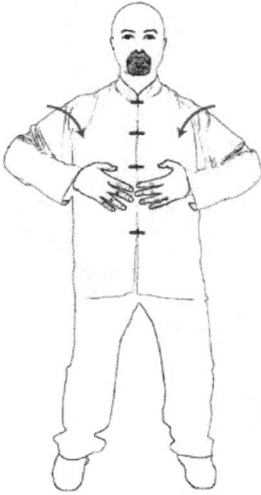

A

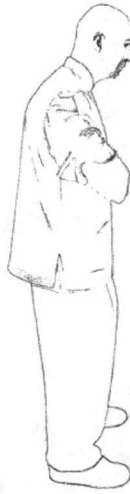

A side

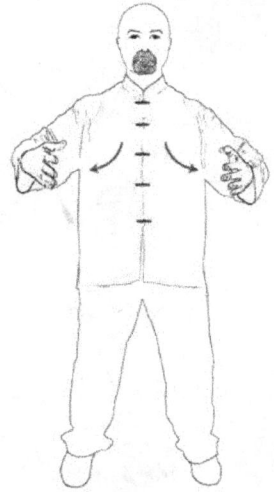

B

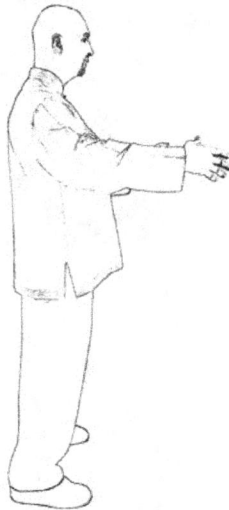

C side

A   Raise arms to the side, circling in front of body, palms facing towards spleen and stomach, between Middle Dan Tian and Lower Dan Tian.

B, C   Move arms away and back from the stomach, no more than body-width, breathing out and letting stale Qi disperse and breathing in, allowing fresh Qi in, three times.

D

E

F

G

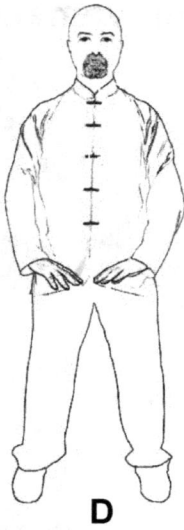

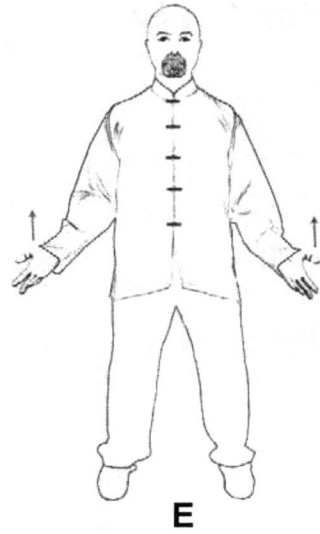

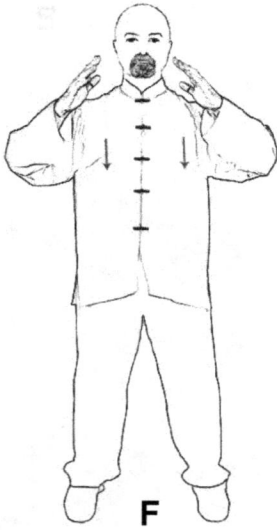

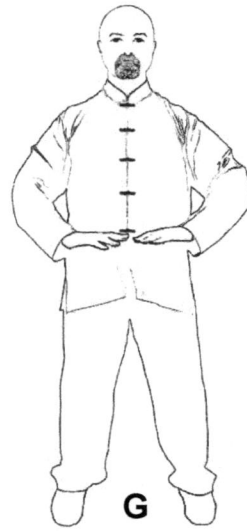

D   Lower the hands in front of the body and separate them at the Dan Tian, fingers pointing down.

E   Raise arms to the side, breathing in, keeping arms down to chest height.

F, G   Again, move the hands down in front of the body and, breathing out (stomach meridian descending) separate at the Dan Tian, fingers pointing down, three times.

Section 2c

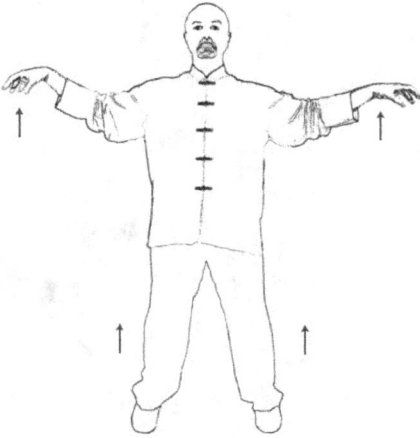

A

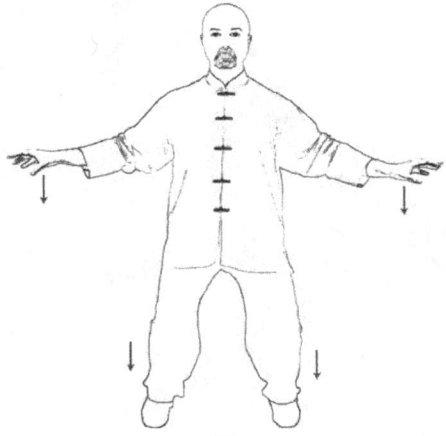

B

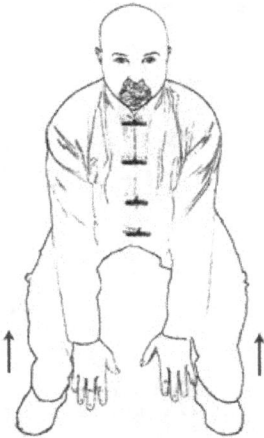

C

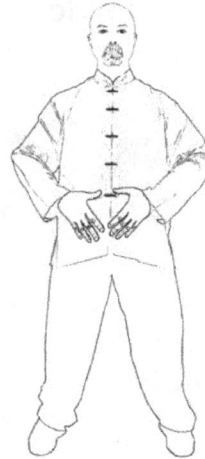

D

A   Raise arms to the side, elbows in and hands holding down floating balls. At the same time, raise and the lower legs in coordination with arms (flying movement) drawing Earth Qi to your hands each time, breathing in.

B, C   Breathing out, bend knees a bit lower and on the third time go as low as you can.

D   Arms spreading around the knees, finger tips facing the ground, push from legs raising arms, palms facing body (Spleen Qi rising up inside leg).

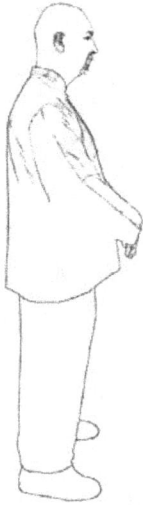

D side

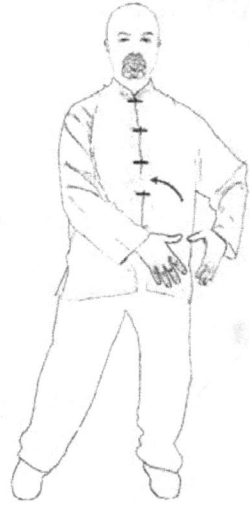

E

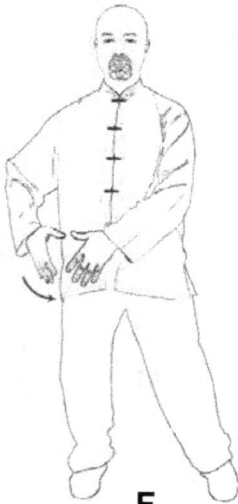

F

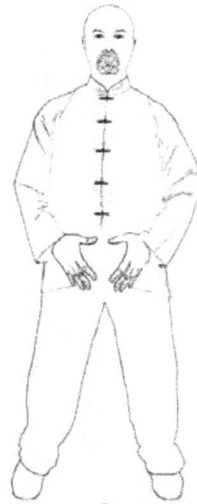

G

E, F,   With palms facing the body, move hands in a clockwise direction
G   three times around the stomach (as if drawing small circles inside),
       and finish on the right side. Then do the movement three times in
       a counter clockwise direction.

Finish on the right hand side, fingers pointing down.

Section 2d

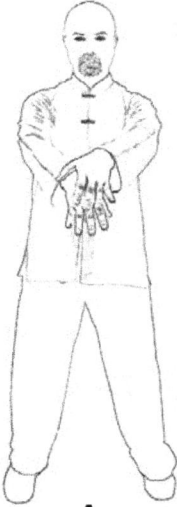

A

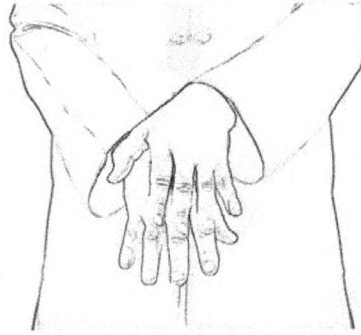

A

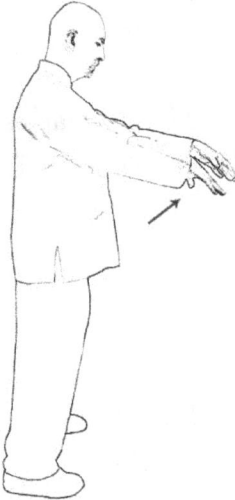

B side

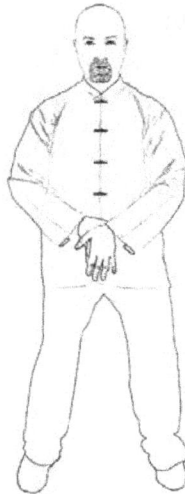

C

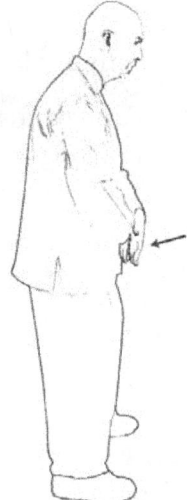

C side

A   Connect the Lao Gong points in the palms of the hands energetically, left hand on top of the right hand about 5cm apart.

B, C   Then move the hands away from the stomach, and then push them back in and together again, thinking of the Qi going towards the spinal bone, three times.

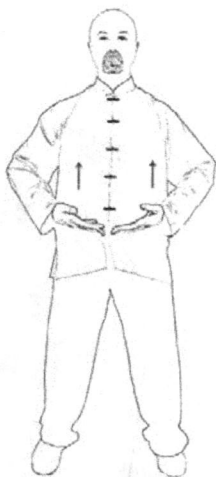 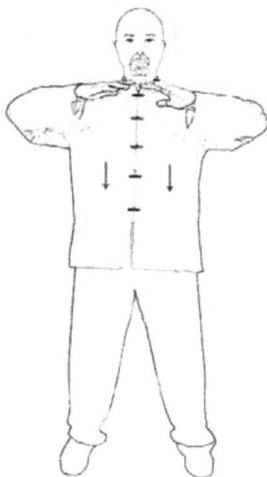 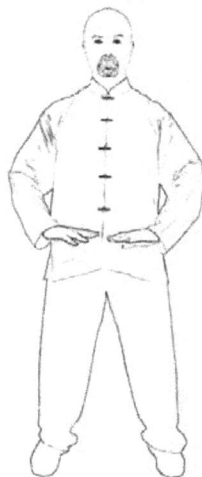

D   **E**   **F**

D   Relax the hands, palms facing up, and raise your hands up to chest height, thinking of your lips (spleen associates with the lips) and letting saliva or Jade Nectar form in the mouth.

E, F   Turn palms to face the ground and swallow Jade Nectar as you slowly guide the hands and Jade Nectar to the Dan Tian and separate, fingers pointing to the ground.

Finish with closing movement

(See instructions page 30)

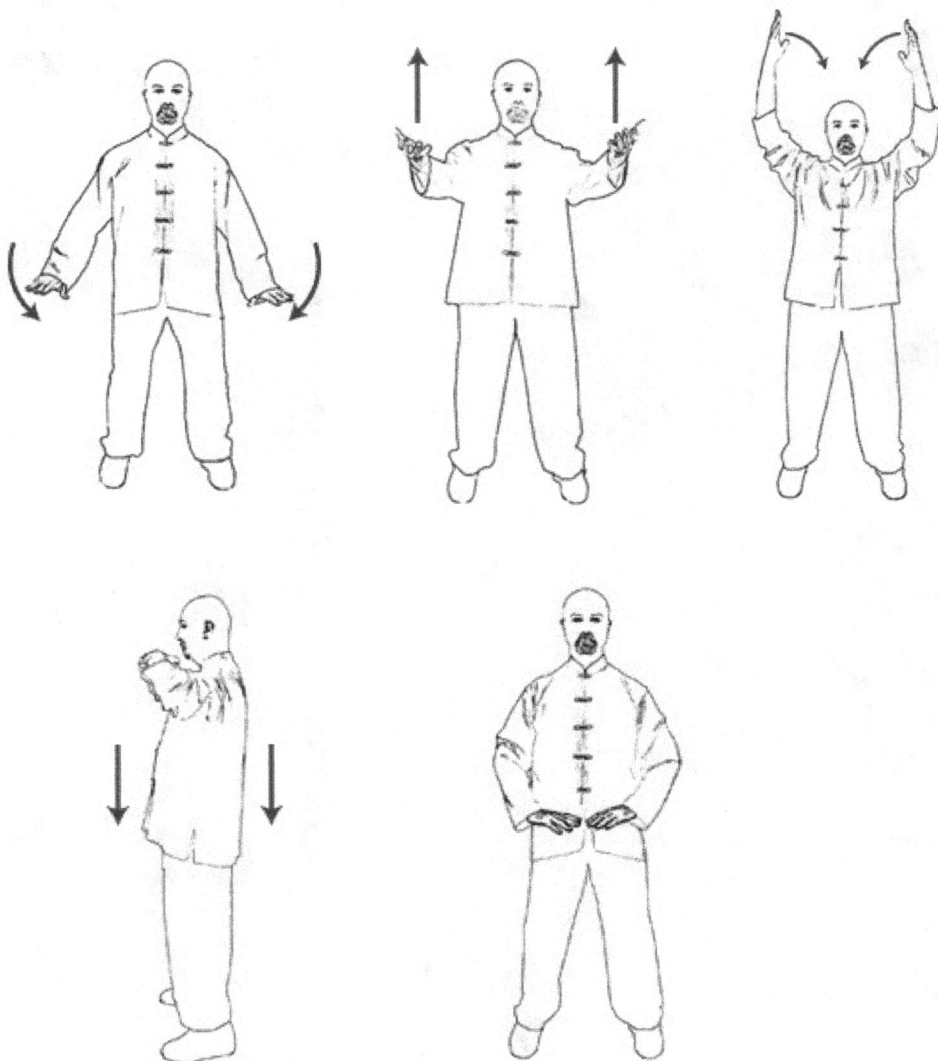

Repeat 3 times.

To close, place hands on the Dan Tian

Just relax, allowing your breath, mind and energy to settle, returning to nothingness.

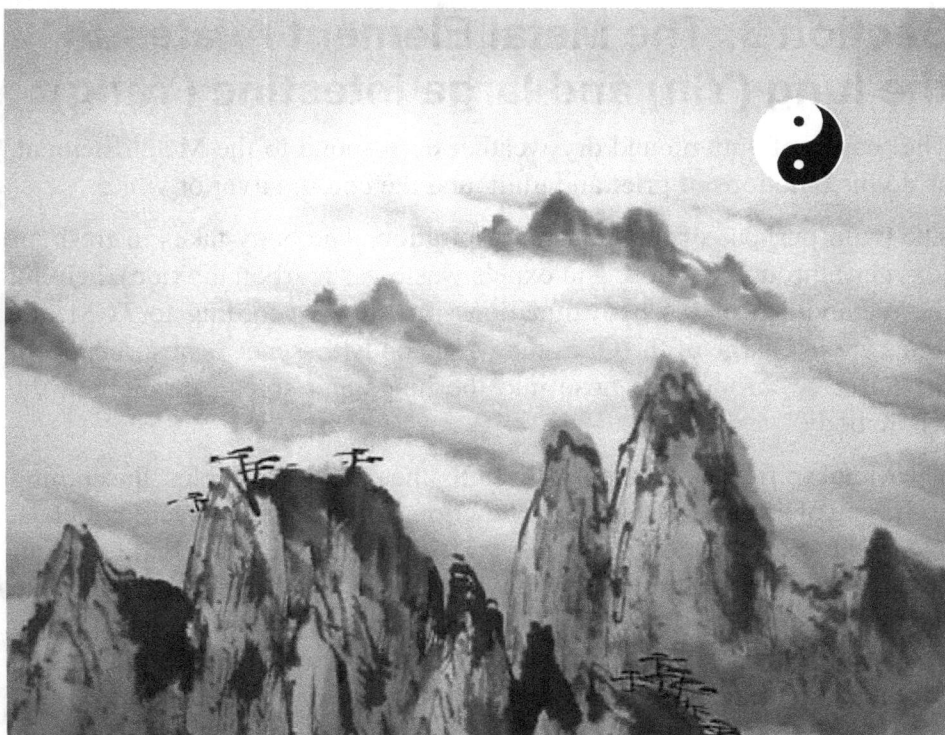

Chapter 7

Section 3: The Metal Element

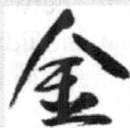

金

Restoring Natural Harmony

Section 3: The Metal Element relates to the lung (Yin) and large intestine (Yang)

The season of autumn and dry weather correspond to the Metal Element, as do the emotions of grief and guilt, and the colour silver or white.

The main purpose of the lungs is respiration. The body takes in fresh air (oxygen) through the nose and expels waste gas (carbon dioxide), helping the metabolism of the body function smoothly. According to TCM, the lungs are in charge of the Qi of the whole body. Essence is absorbed from the universe through the nose into the lungs and spread throughout the whole body.

The Metal spirit is associated with death, the endings of cycles, the coming and going of life, and the excretory functions. Like crystals, precious metals, and minerals, the energy of metal resides deep down, in the depths of our being, the anus and intestines. Metal Qi bestows a deep inner strength, like ore mined from the mountains. A person with well balanced Metal energy is well organised, self disciplined, and conscientious. A person with Metal Qi imbalance may be grief-stricken and steeped in sadness.

The benefits of section 3 described by Dr Xu, "This part is designed to disperse the Qi blocked in arms, lung, nose, heart and chest areas."

The Lung (Yin) channel originates at an area below the collar bone and runs down the inside of the arm to the outside of the thumb. The Large Intestine (Yang) channel originates from the outside of the index finger through the Hegu, or tiger's mouth, between the thumb and index finger along the outside of the arm to the shoulder, to the neck and finishing on the opposite side of the face near the nose and cheek bone.

The Lung Channel

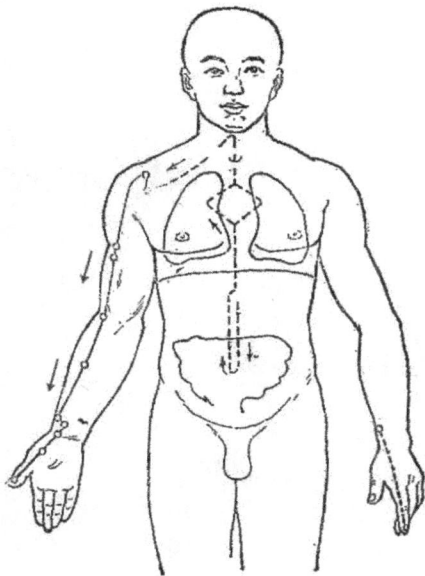

The Large Intestine Channel

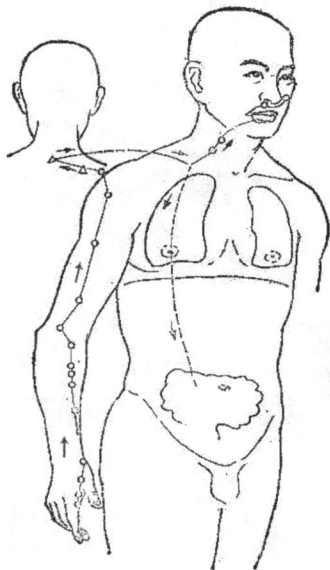

Section 3a: Commencement movement

(See instructions page 30)

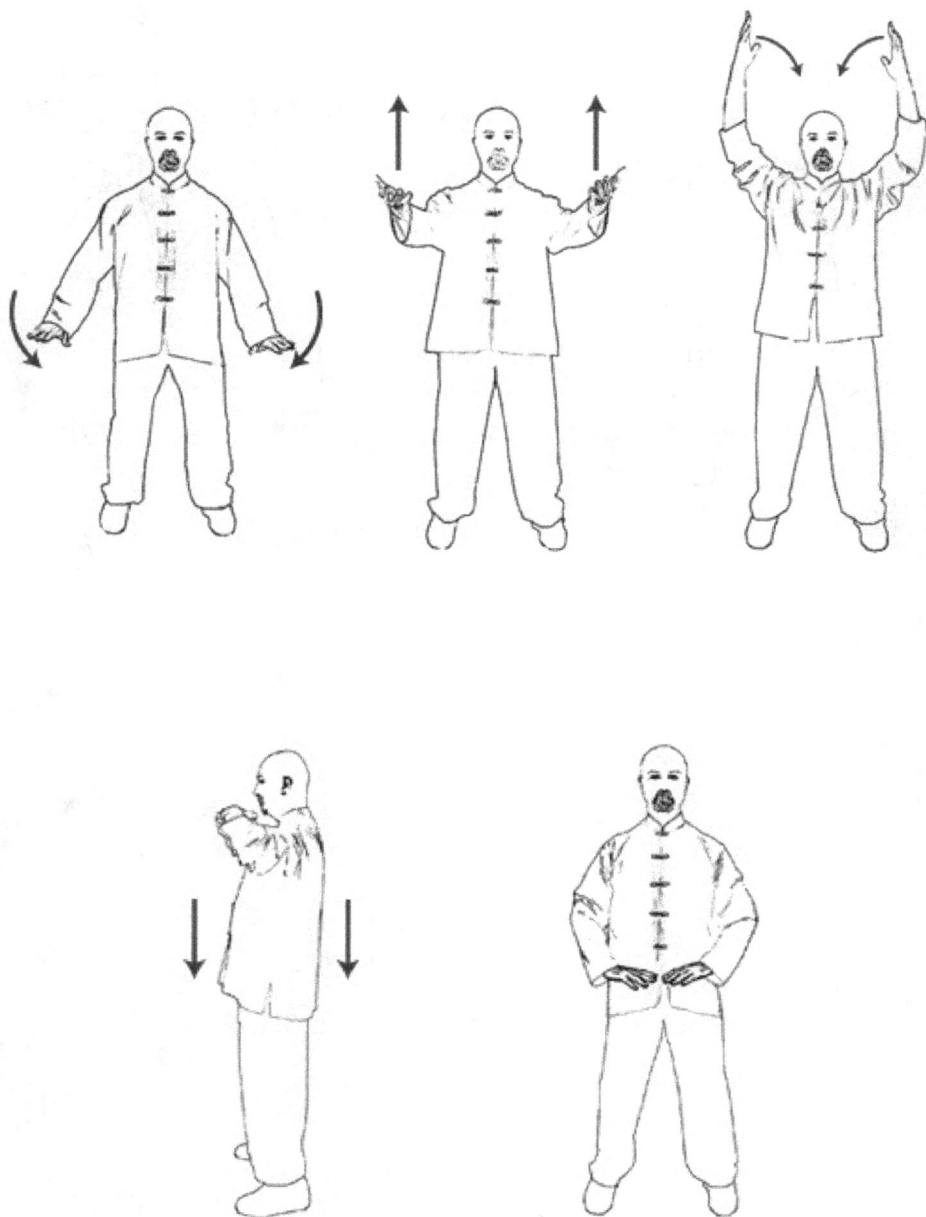

Section 3b: Lung and large intestine movement

Please note that the images are mirrored to the reader; just follow in the same direction.

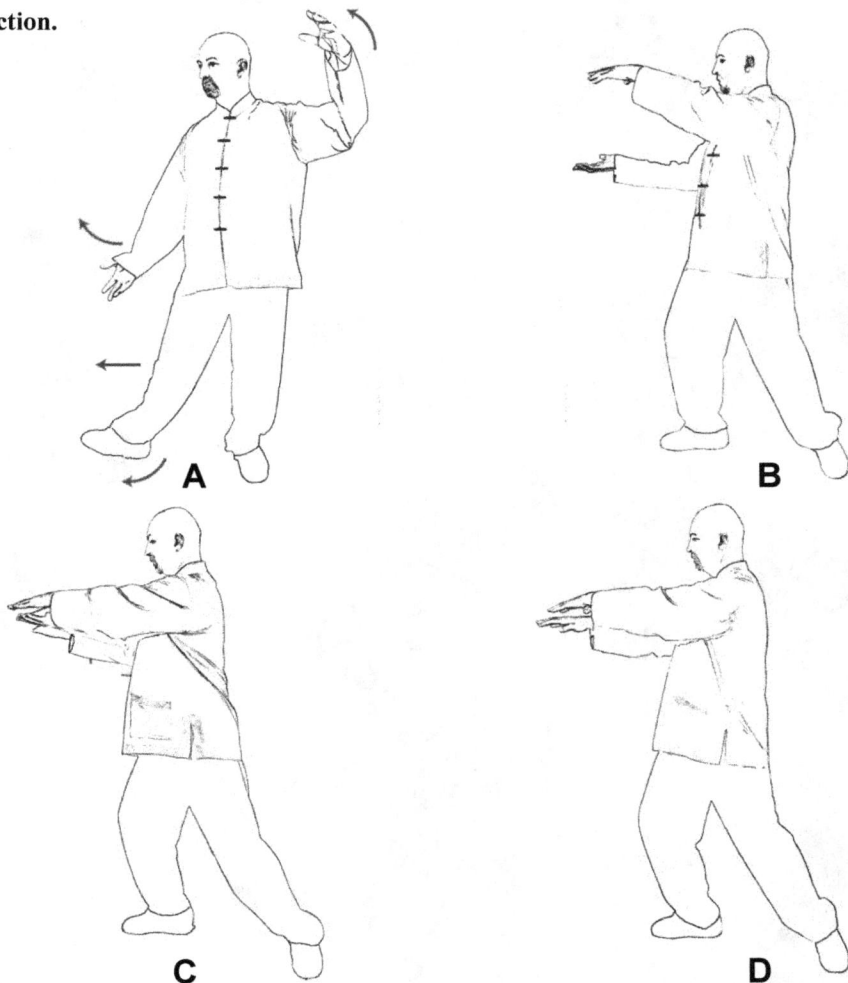

A, B Move the weight 60% to the right. Raise your right arm palm upwards over head and pivot, turning the left toe out 90°. Move your weight 60% over the left leg, raise your left arm to shoulder height and align with the right arm right palm facing down, left palm facing up, holding a ball.

C Feel the Qi between the hands. Note that the right arm must move more quickly than the left arm.

D Rotate the left arm so now the left palm is facing down and feel the Qi on the back of the left hand.

Section 3c

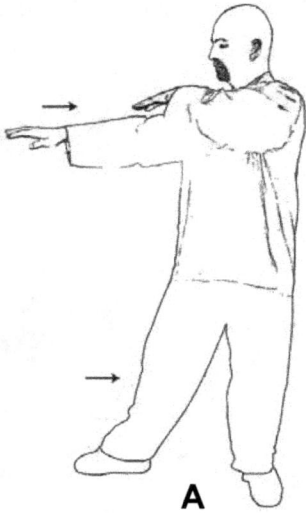

A

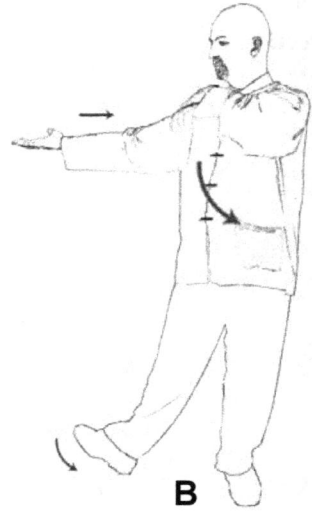

B

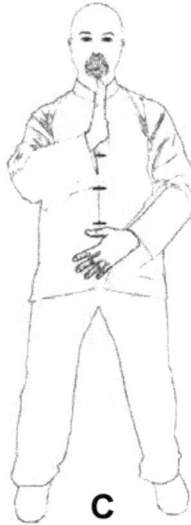

C

A Right palm moves up to shoulder just above left arm along Yang channel (outside arm), fingers pointing forward.

B Rotate the left arm to turn palm up. With elbow down, the left hand moves to the shoulder as the right palm faces the body and moves down in a circle around the lung to middle of body over large intestine.

C Pivoting on the left heel, turn the toe and body to face the front with the left hand in front of the chest below the chin and right palm over the lower abdomen.

Section 3d

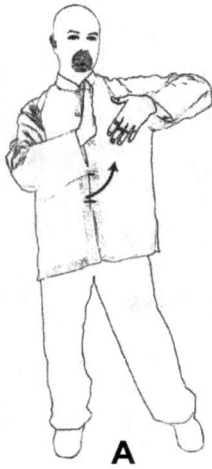

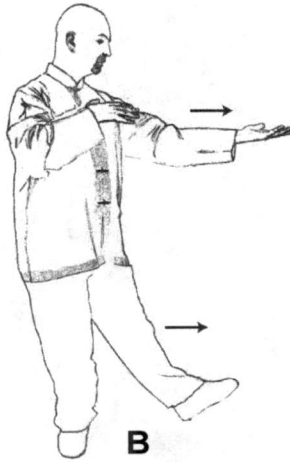

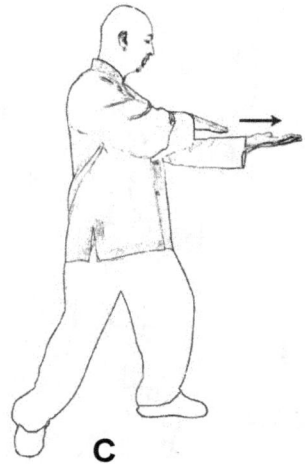

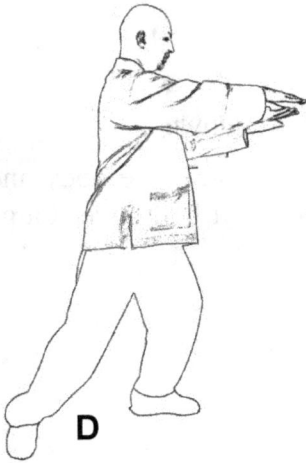

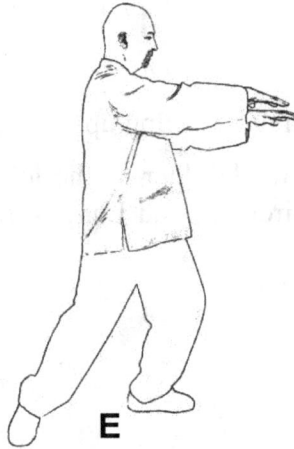

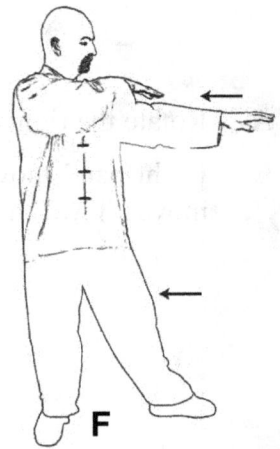

A The right palm continues in a circle following around the lung to the right breast. Pivot on your right heel, turning the right toe out 90°.

B The right arm moves to the top of the right shoulder and unfolds, palm facing up.

C The left hand, palm down, fingers in the direction of the right arm, traces down the right arm following the Yin channel (inside of arm) at the same time moving weight 60% over the right leg.

D, E, Turn right hand over, palm facing down, left palm draws up right
F arm along Yang channel to shoulder, fingers pointing in the direction of the right arm.

Section 3e

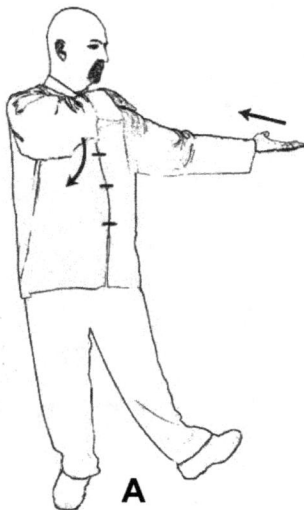

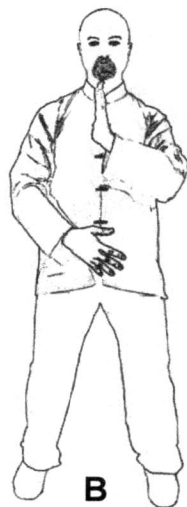

A

B

A   Rotate the right arm palm facing up with elbows down.

B   Right hand moves to shoulder as the left palm faces the body and moves down in a circle around Lung to middle of body over Large Intestine.

Section 3f

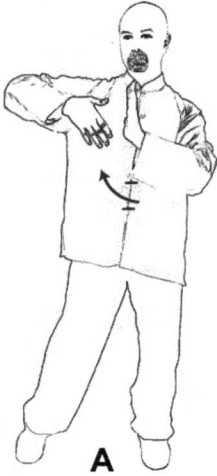

A

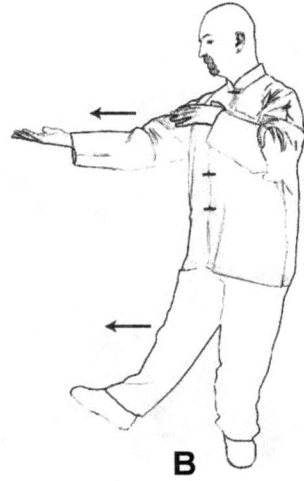

B

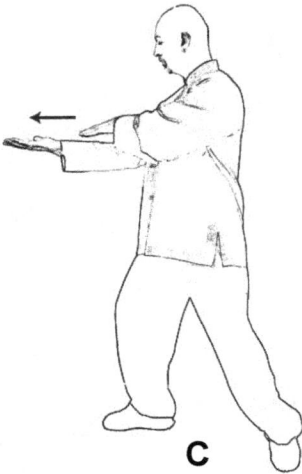

C

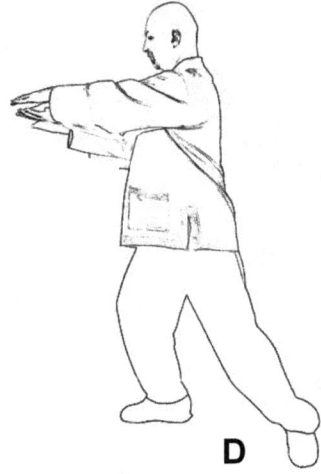

D

A   Pivoting on the right heel, turn toe and body to face the front, right hand in front of the chest under chin and left palm over lower abdomen.

B   Left palm continues in circle following around the Lung to left breast.

C   Pivot on left heel turning left toe out 90°, left arm moves to top of left and unfolds, palm facing up.

D   The right palm traces down left arm following Yin channel, fingers pointing in the direction of the left arm, moving weight 60% over left leg.

Section 3g

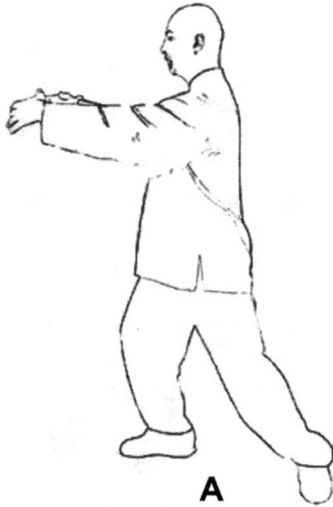

A

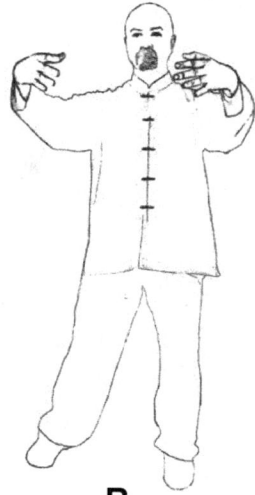

B

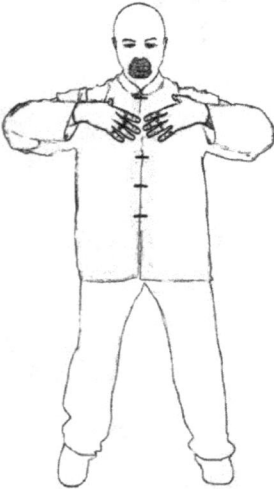

C

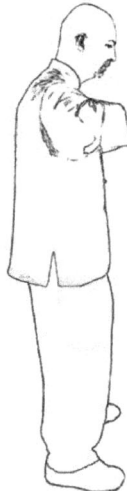

C side

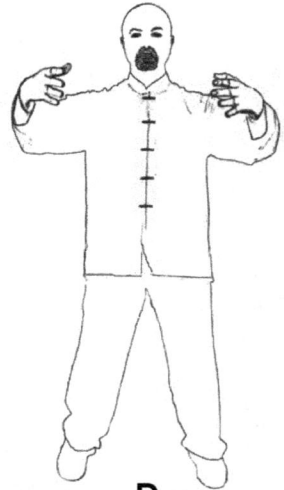

D

A   When reaching the Lao Gong point at the palms, the hands turn 90° to be vertical, arms bending from elbows to body width as if a balloon is expanding, opening the lungs.

B   Pivot on left heel turning toe and body to front.

C, D   With elbows held high move hands in and away from lung and breast, not beyond body width, three times; breathing out hands moving away from lungs allowing the stale Qi out and breathing in hands moving towards lungs letting the fresh Qi in.

Section 3h

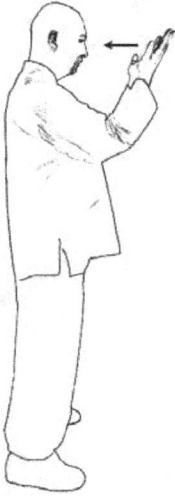

A side

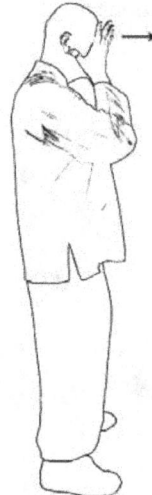

B side

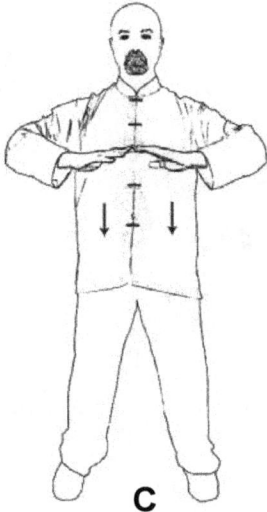

C

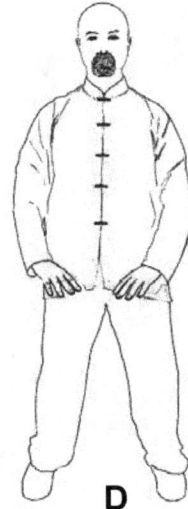

D

A, B Relax elbows in front of torso, palms turn to face the face, Lao Gong point in palms of hands over Large Intestine Acupuncture point between the cheek bone and the nose, moving in and out three times, breathing in moving closer allowing the fresh Qi in and breathing out hands moving away allowing stale Qi out.

C, D Hands move down in front of body, separating at Dan Tian, fingers pointing to ground.

Finish with closing movement

(See instructions page 30)

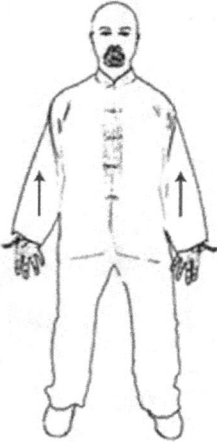

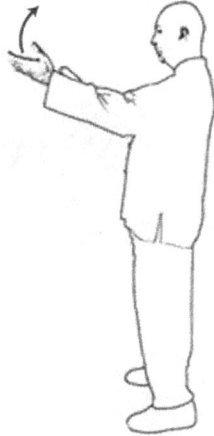

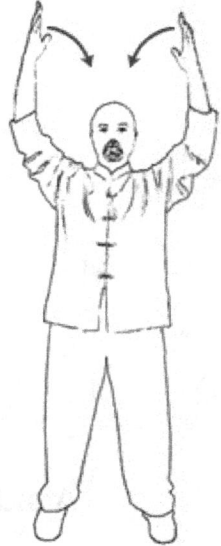

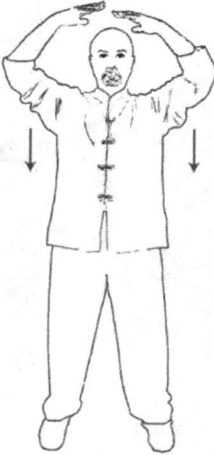

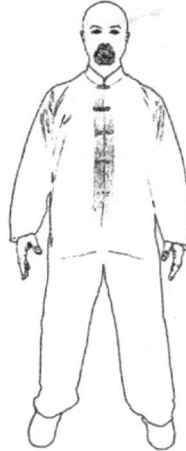

Complete this section again on the other side, starting with the right hand side.

Repeat 3 times to both sides.

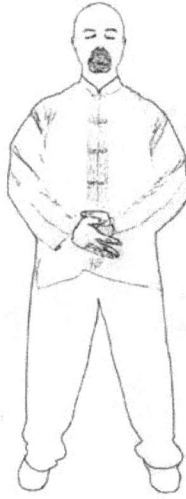

Hands on Dan Tian
Just relax, allowing your breath, mind and energy to settle, returning to nothingness.

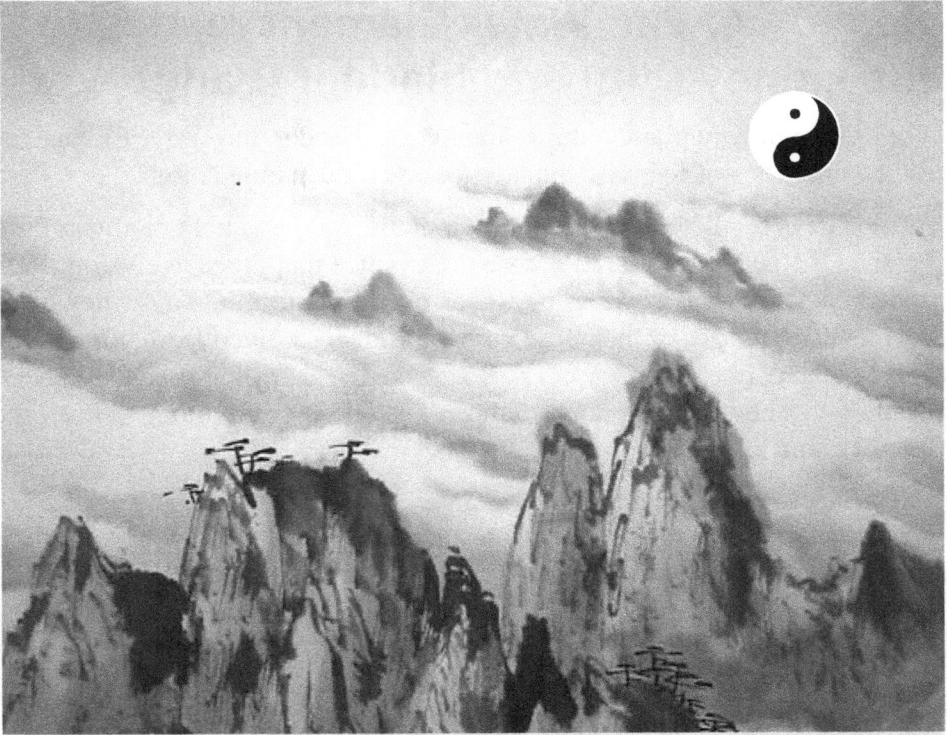

Chapter 8

Section 4: The Water Element

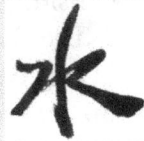

水

Restoring Natural Harmony

Section 4: The Water Element relates to the kidney (Yin) and bladder (Yang)

The season of winter and cold weather correspond to the Water Element as do the emotions of fear and impatience and a deep blue colour.

The kidneys regulate water circulation in the body and help maintain fluid balance. In TCM, the kidneys store the essence that is received from food and air and is released when the other organs require it. Thus, they are a bit like the batteries of the body. Essence is also received from our parents and is stored in the kidneys. The kidneys transform the essence into Qi or energy. They are very important organs and it's important to keep the kidneys warm.

In the macrocosm, the spirit of water can be likened to the power of a hot spring, a geyser that shoots up from the trenches of the deep ocean floor. In the human microcosm it is related to the power of the life force, the instincts, and the driving urgency of ambition. When it is disturbed people continually push themselves to the point of total exhaustion or have no initiative at all. When the Kidney Qi is weak, there can be problems with water metabolism, urination, fertility, or sexuality.

Dr Xu describes the benefits of section 4: "This section can be used for the problems in urinary, reproductive organs, back and lower back pain, problems in the ear and head."

The Kidney channel (Yin) originates from the sole of the foot, Yongquan, and rises around the ankle up the inside of the leg, through the abdomen to the chest below the collar bone. The Bladder channel (Yang) originates from an area near the eyebrow, just off centre and goes back over the head, descends down the back to the hip area, continues down the back of the legs to the heel, along the outside of the foot finishing on the outside of the small toe.

The Kidney Channel

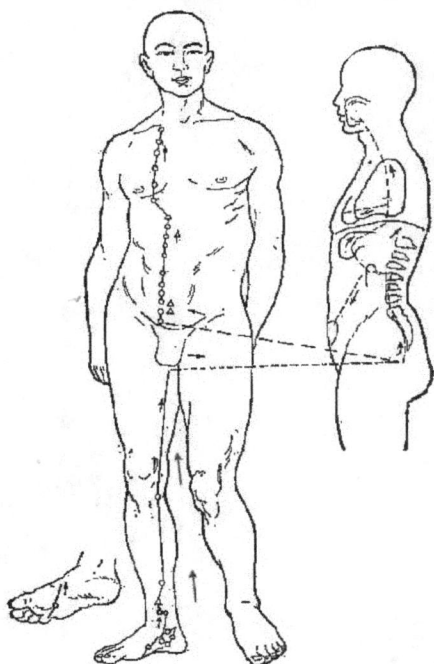

The Urinary Bladder Channel

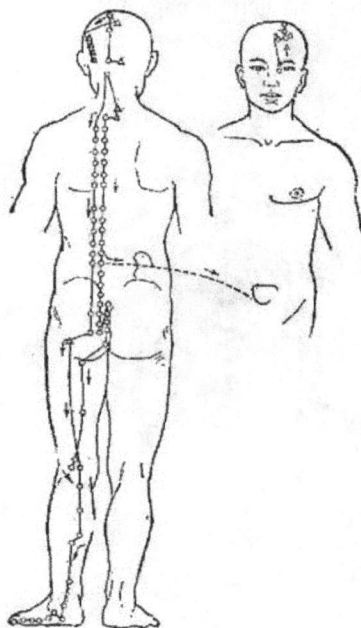

Section 4a: Commencement movement
(See instructions page 30)

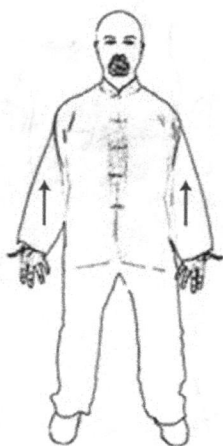

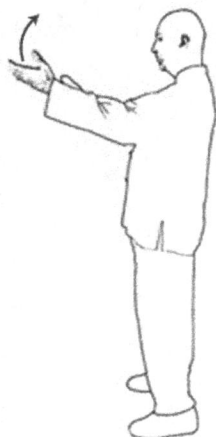

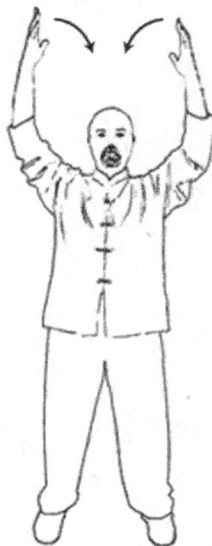

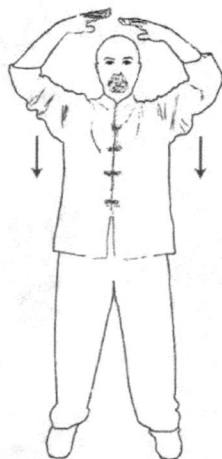

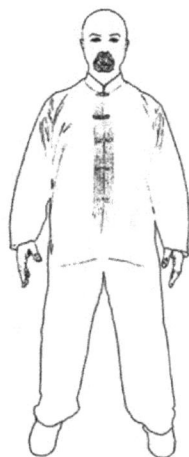

Section 4b: Kidney and bladder movement

Please note that the images are mirrored to the reader; just follow in the same direction.

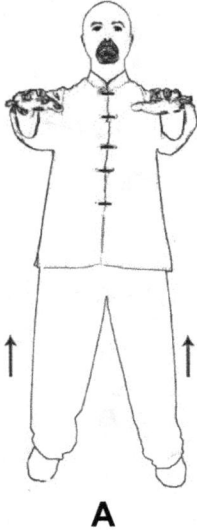

A

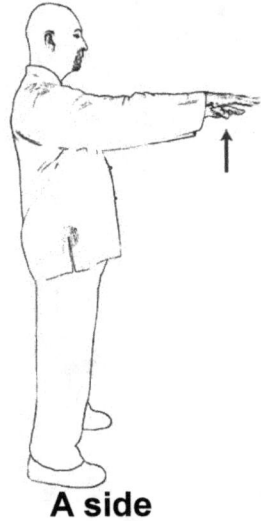

A side

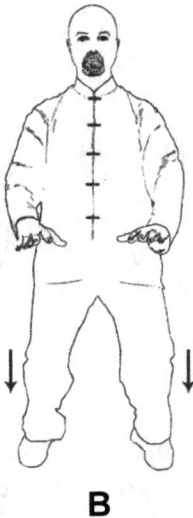

B

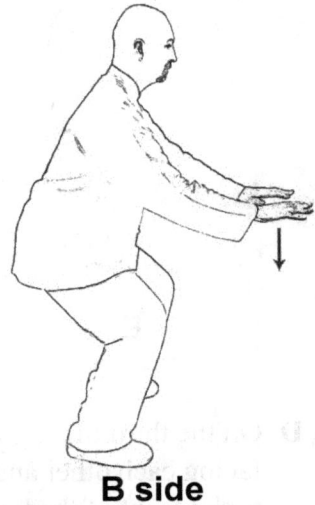

B side

A   Raise arms to shoulder height, palms facing the ground.

B   Lower your arms in coordination with the knees until hands reach navel height. Raise up to full height and down again two more times, each time bending the knees to go a little bit lower.

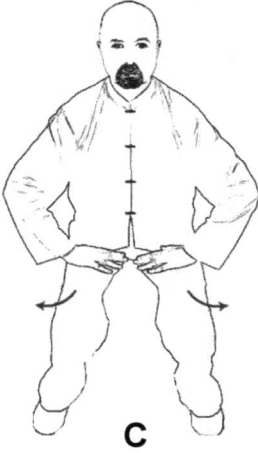

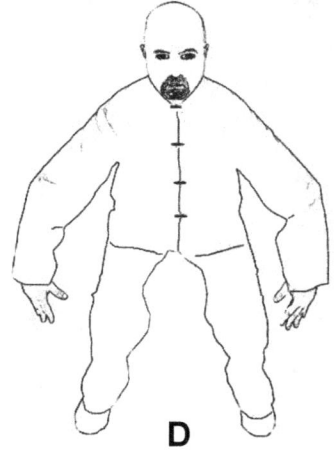

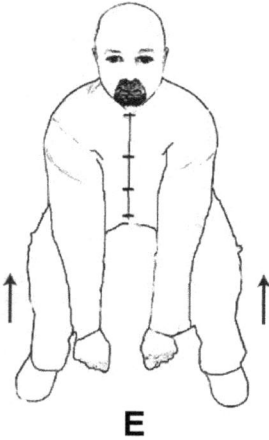

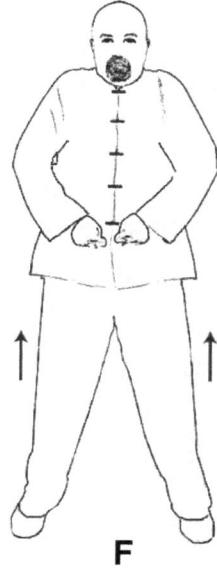

C, D On the third time, go as low as is comfortable, turn hands in, fingers facing each other and push hands to the side over your knee, circling to the front of the body.

E, F Clenching fists with thumbs on the inside, grip toes, tense legs, hold up Hui Yin (pelvic floor), clench teeth, lift shoulders, tense whole body but (importantly) only about 30% to 40%. Push from legs and raise hands to navel height (like lifting a heavy weight).

Section 4c

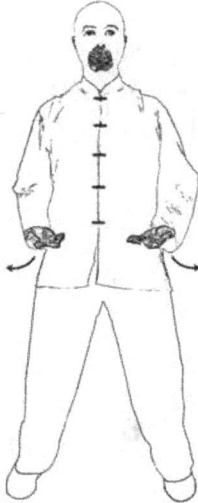

A

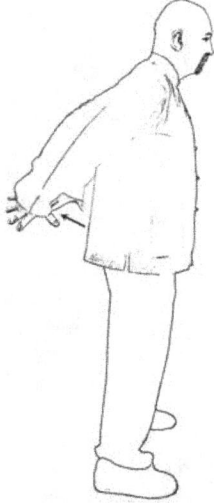

B Side

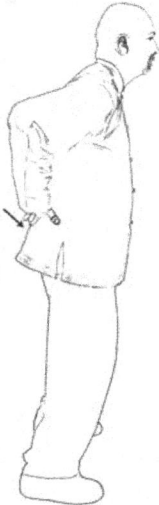

C Side

A   Palms turn up as they draw back around the belt channel (waist); relax hands and whole body as hands pass hips.

B, C Palms facing kidney area moving hands in and away three times, breathing out allowing stale Qi out and breathing in, letting fresh Qi in.

Section 4d

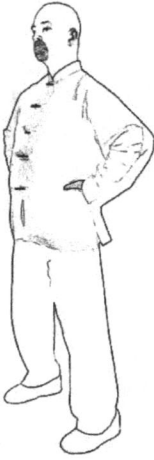

A

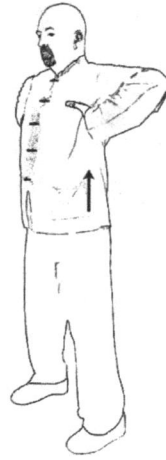

B

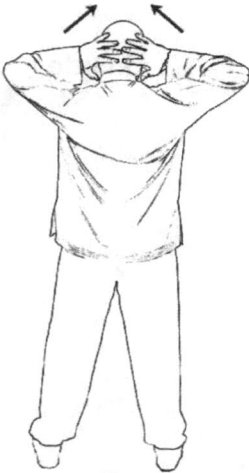

C rear

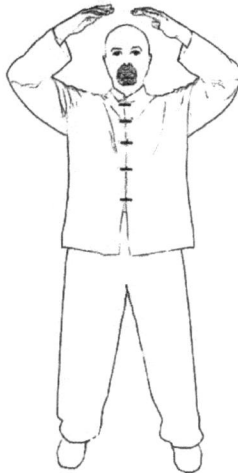

D

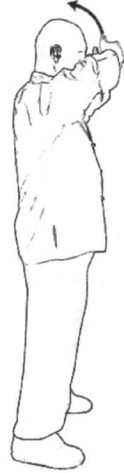

E side

A   Palms facing up with thumbs pointing forward, tense whole body, grip toes, tense legs, hold up Hui Yin (pelvic floor), clench teeth, lift shoulders, again only about 30% to 40%.

B   Raise palms up side of body, breathing in, brushing the surface of skin to under arms then circle around chest to back of neck, breath out and relax whole of body.

C, D,   Palms facing base of skull circle over head to forehead, palms
E   about 5cm from head, back and forward three times, stimulating bladder channel.

Section 4e

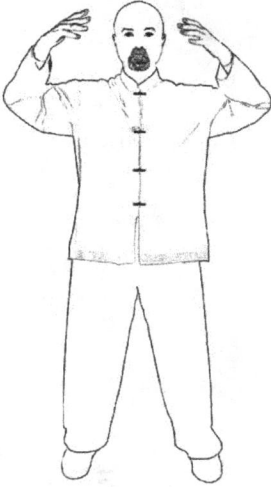

A

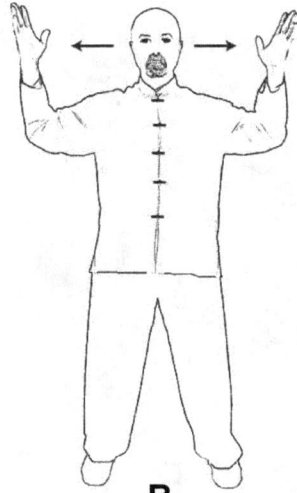

B

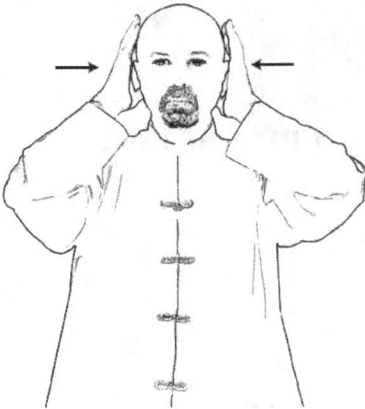

C

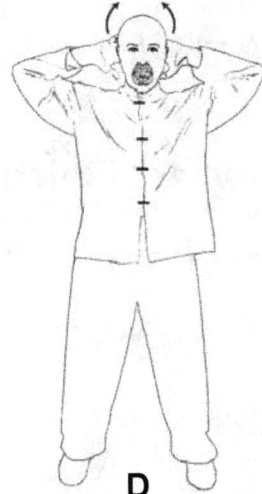

D

A   Separate hands in front of forehead while looking into the distance like opening a door (opening the third eye).

B, C   Hands move in and away from ear three times (Qi from Lao Gong through ear canal to middle of the head).

D   Palms move to base of skull, circle over head to forehead.

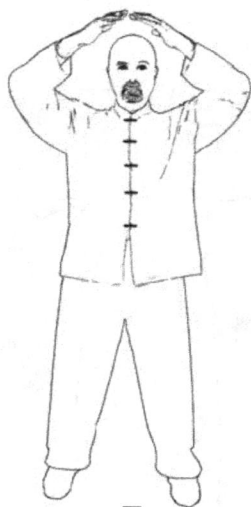

E

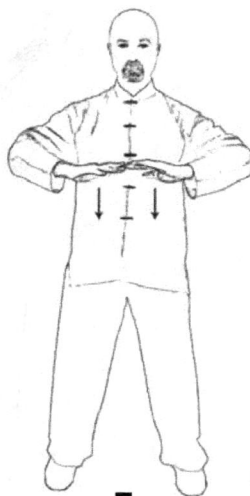

F

E, F Hands move down in front of body separating at Dan Tian, fingers pointing to ground.

Section 4e: Finish with closing movement
(See instructions page 30)

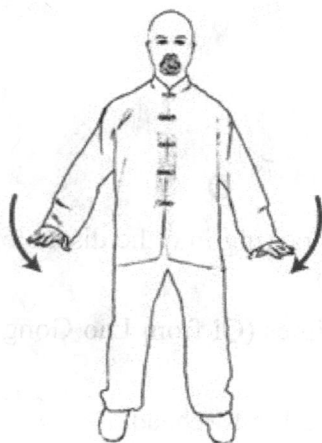

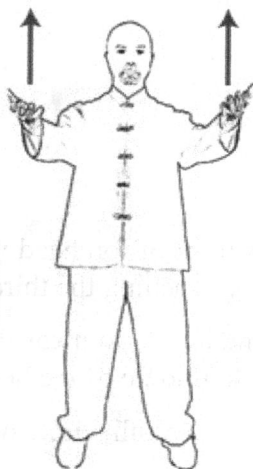

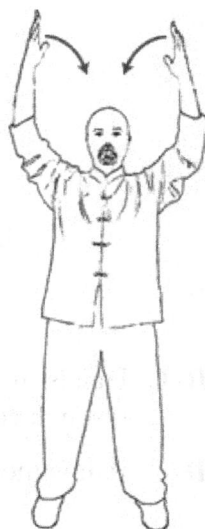

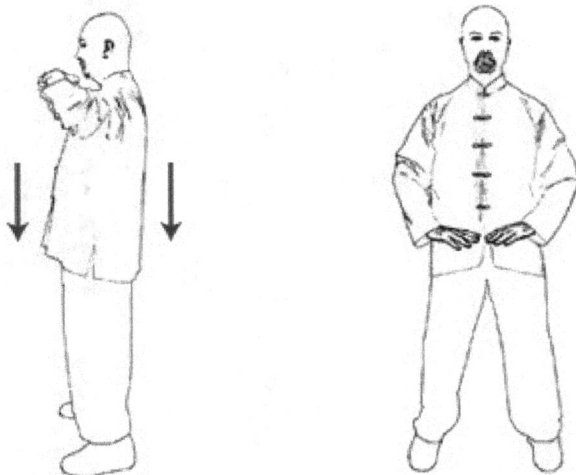

Repeat 3 times.

Hands on Dan Tian

Just relax, allowing your breath, mind and energy to settle, returning to nothingness.

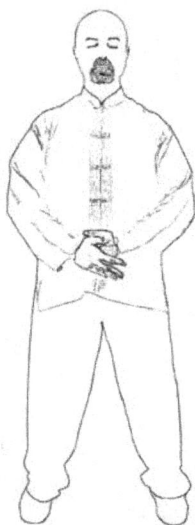

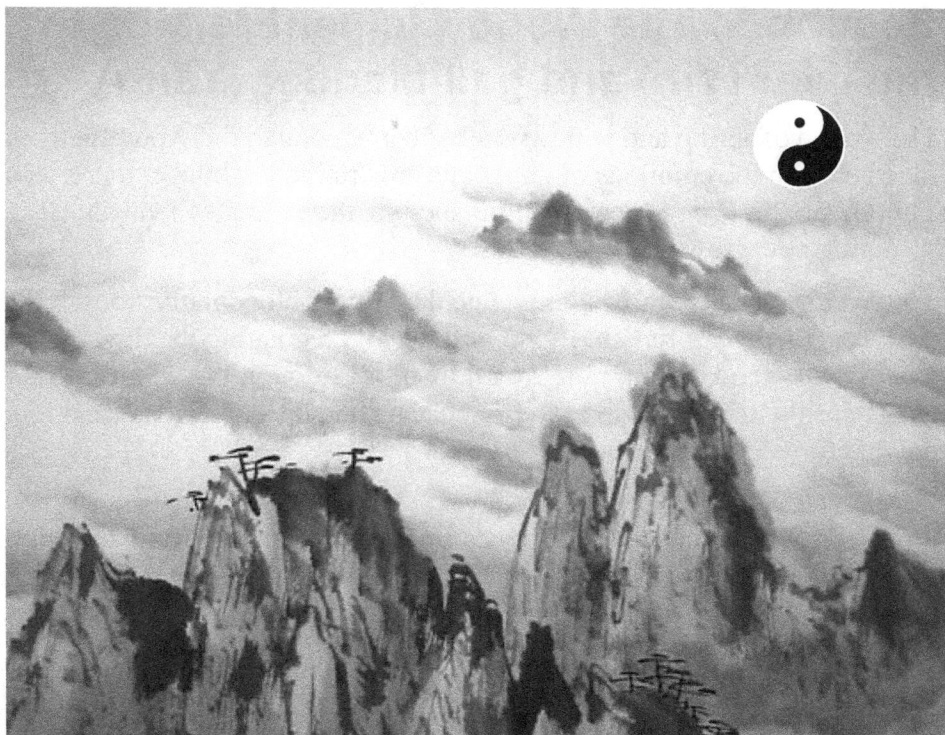

Chapter 9

Section 5: The Wood Element

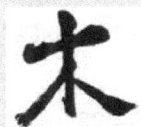

木

Restoring Natural Harmony

Section 5: The Wood Element relates to the liver (Yin) and gall bladder (Yang)

The season of spring and windy weather correspond to the Wood Element, together with the emotions of anger and frustration, and the colour green. The Qi of the Wood element flourishes in the spring when plants are sprouting new growth.

The liver helps to cleanse and regulate the flow of blood in the body. TCM describes the liver's function as smoothing and regulating the flow of vital energy and blood, helping the free flow of Qi through the whole body. It also helps the spleen to send food essence up and the stomach to send food down, normalising digestion.

People with strong Wood energy have a clear vision and goals, and know how to bring them into being. They excel at decision making and planning. With the spirit of wood we see form beginning to emerge from formlessness with clear direction and imagination. Wood energy maintains the balance of emotional life.

When the wood Qi is weak, people can be indecisive and 'stuck' in life. They may be constrained emotionally, unable to express anger. If the emotions are repressed, the Qi of the liver will back up and stagnate. This can cause digestive problems like bloating, gas, alternating constipation and diarrhea. The Liver and Gallbladder channels run across the top and sides of the head, common sites for migraine headaches.

The benefits of section 5 described by Dr Xu: "This part can be used for problems in the arms and shoulders, depression, problems in the head and eye, liver and gallbladder."

The Liver channel (Yin) originates from the big toe moves around the ankle and rises up the inside into the body past the hip, finishing at the lower rib area. The Gall Bladder channel (Yang) originates from an area at the outer corner of the eye, runs around the ear, over the side of the head, down the neck to the shoulder, underneath the shoulder and down the side of the body past the hip, descending down the outside of the leg to the ankle along the outside of the foot and finishing at the outside of the fourth toe,

The Liver Channel

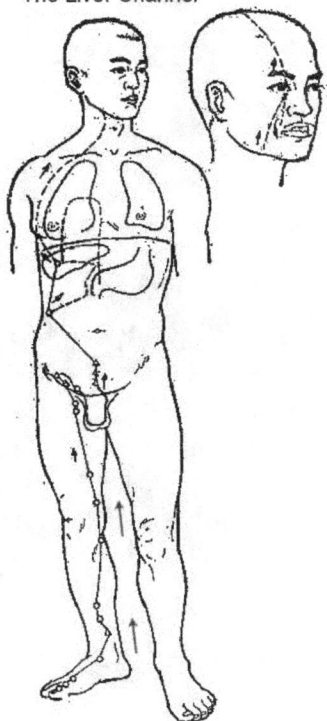

The Gall Bladder Channel

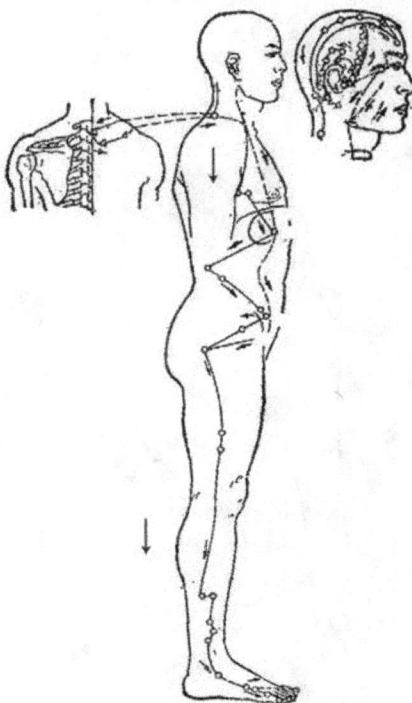

Section 5a: Commencement movement

(See instructions page 30)

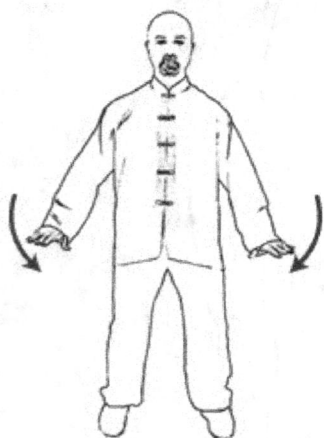

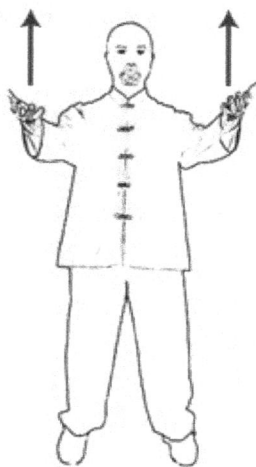

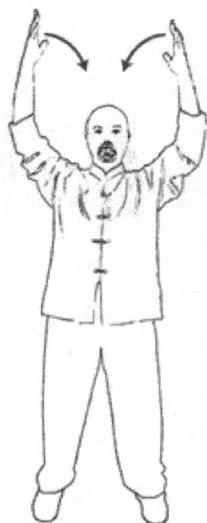

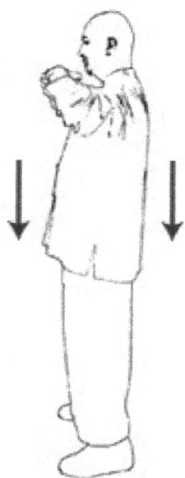

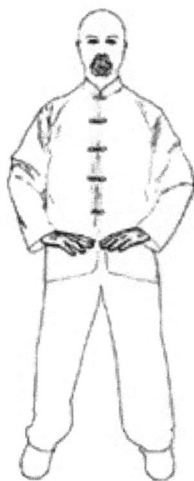

Section 5b: Liver and gall bladder movement

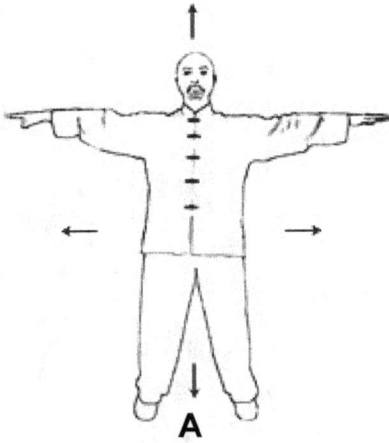

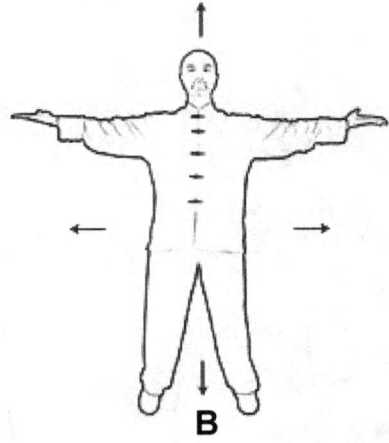

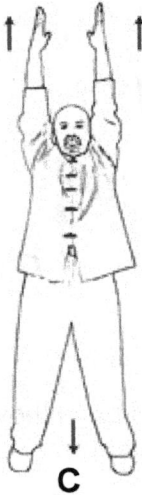

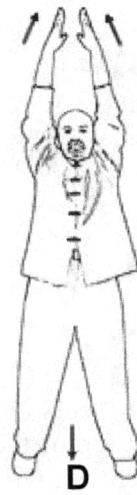

A Arms rise to the side to shoulder height, palms facing the ground, fingers pointing straight. Stretch deliberately and with intention, connecting to the horizon (the property of wood is to expand). Let the stale Qi out as you stretch like a growing tree; hold the stretch for two to three seconds, breathing normally.

B Turn palms up and stretch again for two to three seconds, arms straight.

C Lift shoulders, fingers pointing to the sky (like a tree reaching to the heavens); stretch two to three seconds, again breathing normally.

D Lift heels off the ground, arms tapering in like a pine tree (not touching), and stretch two to three seconds.

Section 5c

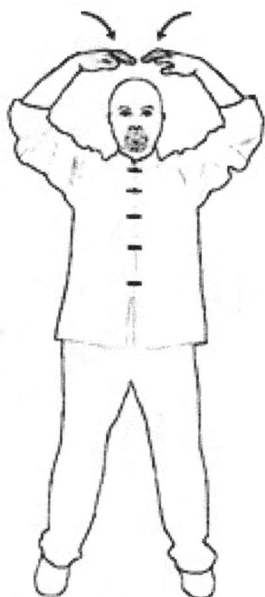

A

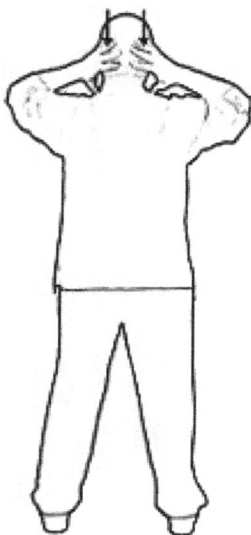

B rear

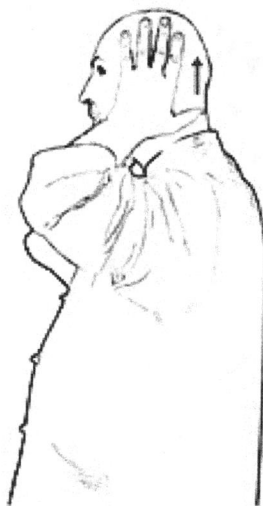

C side

A   Lower heels to the ground, relax the arms, bending elbows, fingers to the top of the head (Bai Hui point) bringing down the heavenly Qi, sending Qi to the Gall Bladder.

B, C   Both palms move down the back of the head and circle around the back of the ears (Gall Bladder points) up the side of the head and over the top again three times.

Section 5d

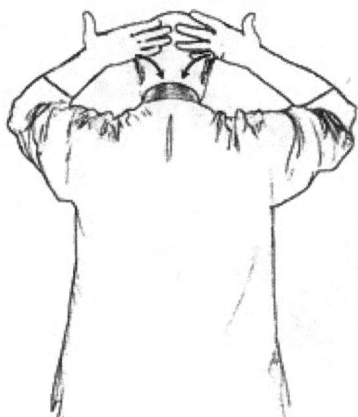

A rear

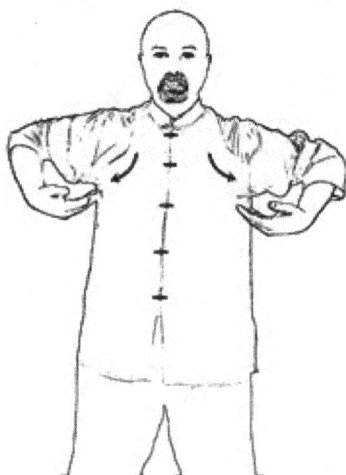

B

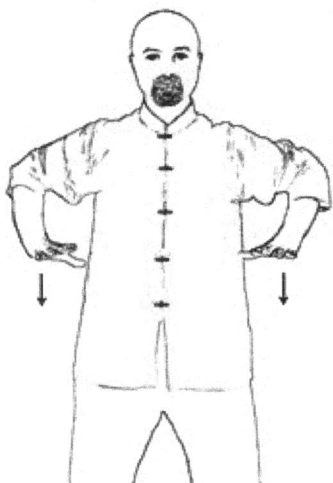

C

A, B   After the third rotation, when hands reach the back of the skull, turn palms out, brushing down neck and under shoulder.

C   Fingers pointing forward and palms facing the ground, open tiger's mouth, and push palms down the sides of the body (Gall Bladder channel) to mid thigh, lowering knees in coordination.

Section 5e

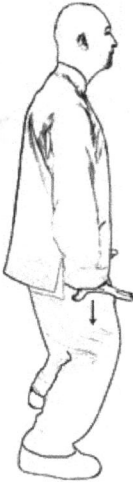

A side

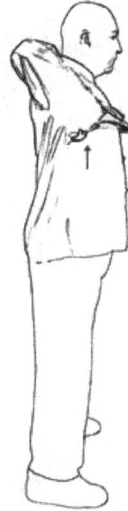

B side

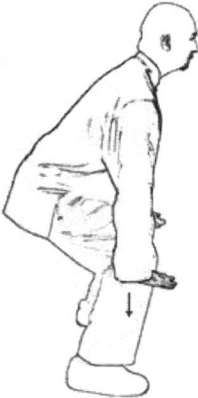

C side

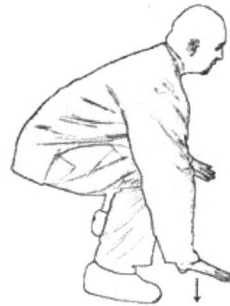

D side

A, B   Raise knees, palms up under armpits, lifting elbows to the side (opening Gall Bladder area).

C   The second time, push right down to below the knee, again raising the knees and arms, opening Gall Bladder area.

D   On the third time, go as low as you can, palms stretching out. Each time, think of Qi going down the legs, like roots of the tree spreading into the earth.

Section 5f

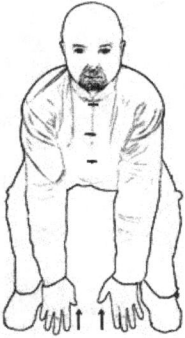

A

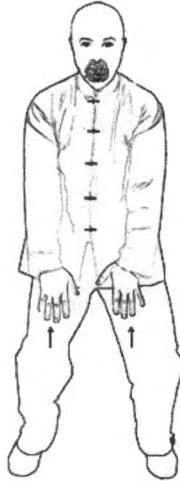

B

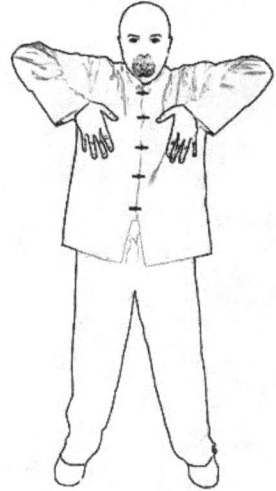

C

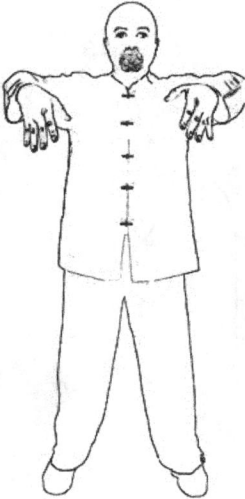

D

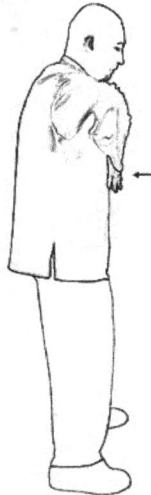

E side

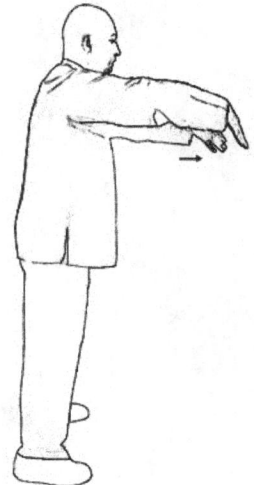

F side

A, B Circle arms around knees, fingers pointing to the ground, and push from the legs raising the body, palms drawing up inside legs, past the hips up the front of the body, tracing the Liver channel (Qi rising to Liver).

C Lift elbows high, like cow horns (opening Gall Bladder area).

D, E, F Move palms in and away three times over the liver on both sides, breathing out as hands move away from the body, allowing stale Qi out, and breathing in as hands move towards the body, letting fresh Qi in.

Section 5g

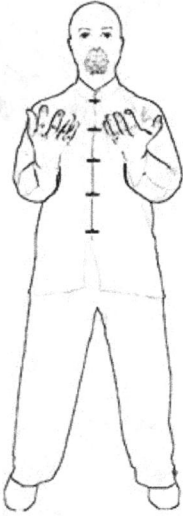

A

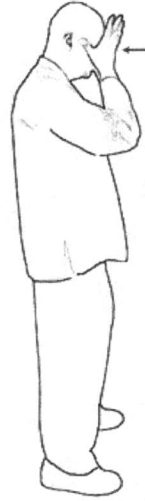

B side

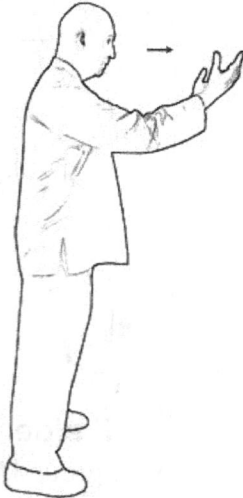

C side

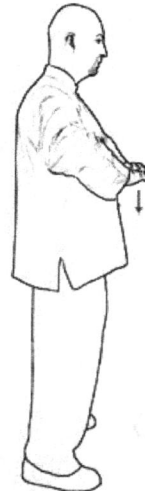

D side

A, B Lower the elbows turn palms up in front of the face (Lao Gong
C to eyes) move in and away three times, breathing in coming closer
and breathing out moving away, looking at palms.

D Hands move down in front of body, separating at Dan Tian,
fingers pointing to ground.

Finish with closing movement
(See instructions page 30)

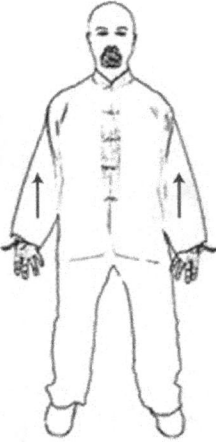

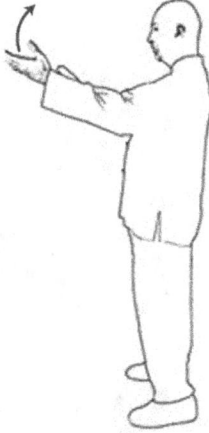

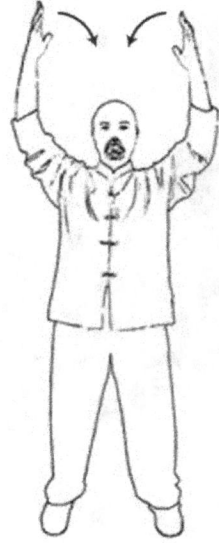

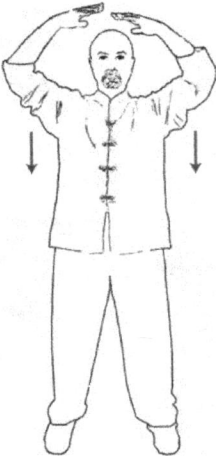

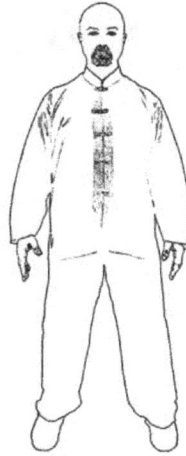

Repeat 3 times.

Hands on Dan Tian

Just relax, allowing your breath, mind and energy to settle, returning to nothingness.

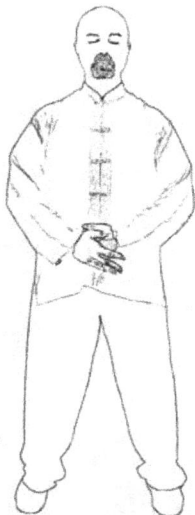

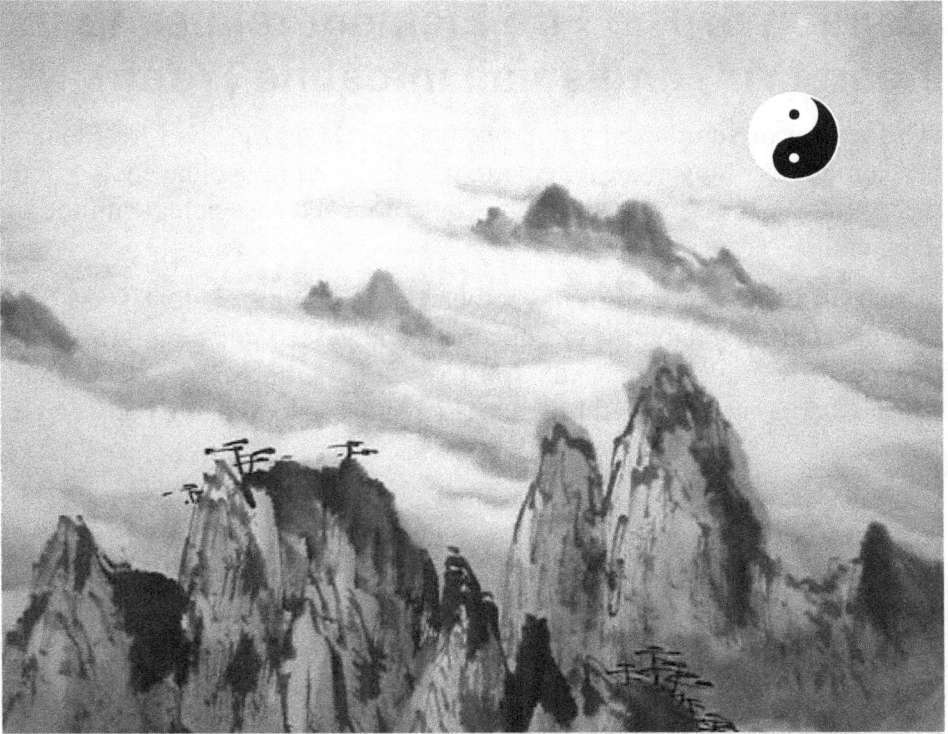

Chapter 10

Section 6: The Fire Element

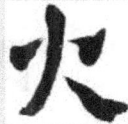

火

Restoring Natural Harmony

Section 6: The Fire Element relates to the heart (Yin) and small intestine (Yang)

The season of summer and hot weather correspond to the Fire Element. The emotions of joy and excitement, which can stimulate the energy of the heart but in excess, can exhaust it. The colour red associates with the fire element.

The heart is the Emperor of the body according to the ancient TCM texts. It propels the blood to flow through the blood vessels and circulate through the body. It is also where the spirit resides. If the Emperor is in good spirits, harmony prevails throughout the whole kingdom, the body and the universe.

During our life, the spirit of fire resides in the centre of the heart, where it continues to grow as it guides us along our path through life. Its presence is reflected in the brightness of our eyes and disposition. When the heart is disturbed by emotion, it is like a turbulent sea. If we can detach from the emotions as they pass, the heart will grow calm again like water after a storm. When the Fire Qi is weak, a person may be lacklustre or bland. They may suffer from anxiety, restlessness, and insomnia.

Fire spirit shines from the heart of a young child as joy and delight, from an adolescent as romance and intellectual curiosity, and with maturity, transforms into the illumination of self-awareness and intuitive knowing.

Dr Xu describes the benefits of section 6: "This section can be used for problems in arms and shoulders, depression, heart, and lung conditions."

The Heart channel (Yin) originates from the centre of the armpit to the bicep, past the elbow to the outside of the wrist finishing at the end of the small finger. The Pericardium channel (Yin), which also relates to the Heart channel, starts next to the nipple and also flows down to the centre of the inside of the arm, finishing at the middle finger. The Small Intestine channel (Yang) starts from the outside tip of the little finger and runs upward along the outside of the arm through the wrist and elbow to the shoulder, then to the neck and cheek and finishes near the ear, at the depression created when the mouth is opened.

The Heart Channel

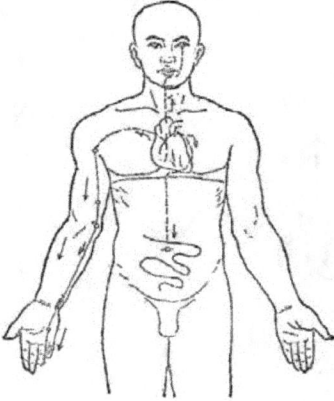

The Pericardium Channel

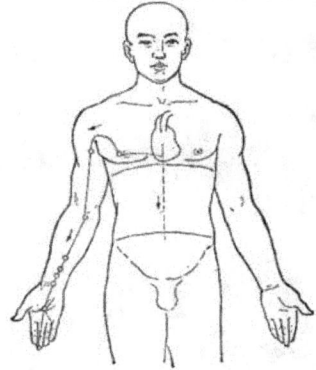

The Small Intestine Channel

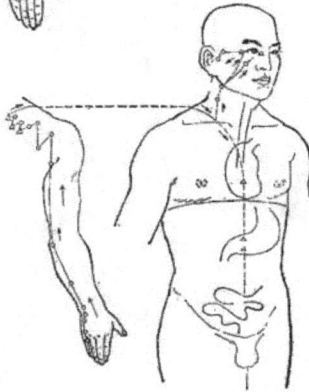

Section 6a: Commencement movement

(See instructions page 30)

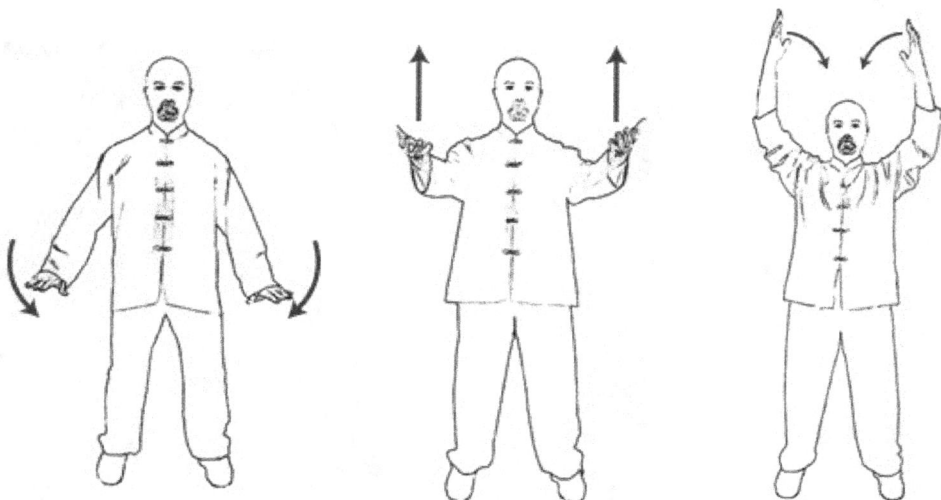

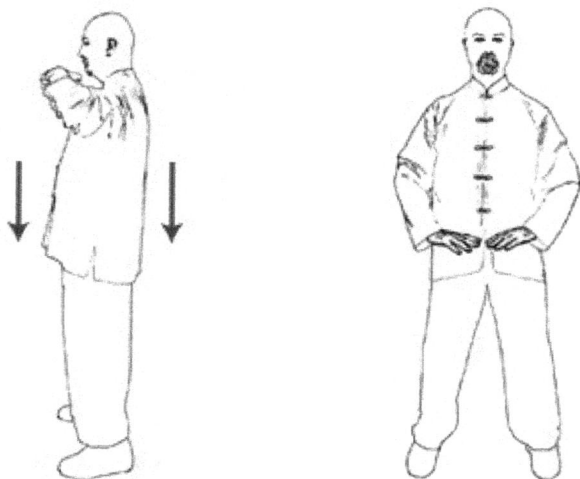

Section 6b: Heart and small intestine movement

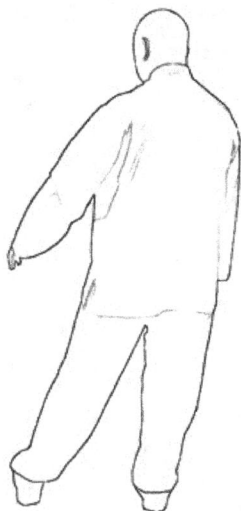 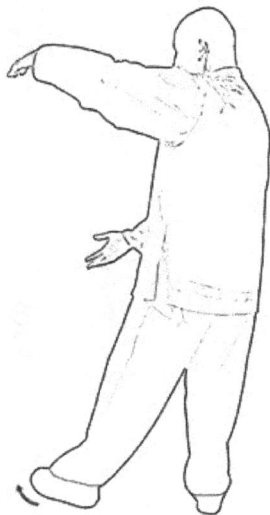 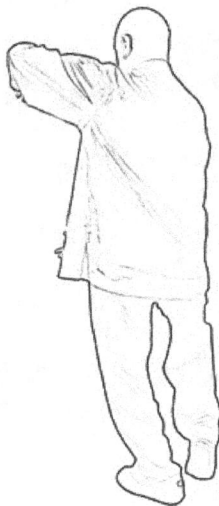

A rear   **B rear**   **C rear**

A   Move body weight over your <u>right</u> leg, turning the <u>left</u> toe out 45°.

B   <u>Left</u> arm sweeps over with the palm facing ground as the <u>right</u> arm sweeps under, palm facing up (holding a large ball).

C   At the same time, move your weight 100% over the <u>left</u> leg, stepping up on <u>right</u> toe.

Section 6c

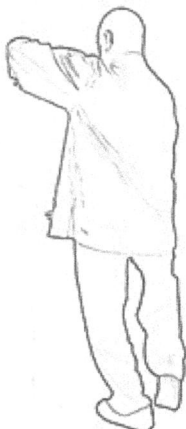

A rear

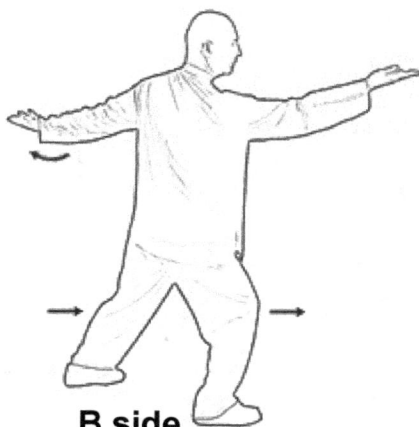

B side

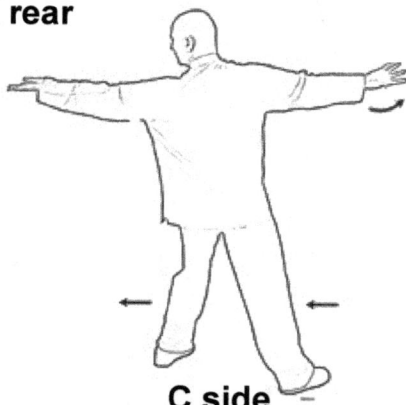

C side

A   <u>Right</u> leg steps forward, moving body weight over <u>right</u> foot as <u>right</u> arm sweeps forward, palm facing up at shoulder height above <u>right</u> foot, fingers pointing forward.

B   The <u>left</u> arm sweeps back, palm facing up at shoulder height, fingers pointing back. Hold the arms in a straight, horizontal line through the arm facing forward, palm up, across the shoulders, to the arm facing back, palm down.

C   Looking forward, push from front leg back, rotating both arms and turning the head, following from palm twisting across shoulders to the back arm, palm facing up, finish with weight over <u>left</u> leg (60%). Move back and forward three times, twisting and stretching and turning the palms to stretch the Heart and Small Intestine channels, bringing warmth to the heart and chest each time as if a ball of fire (the sun) rolls from one palm to the other, with the eyes and head following.

Finish with 100% body weight over the <u>left</u> leg, looking back.

Section 6d

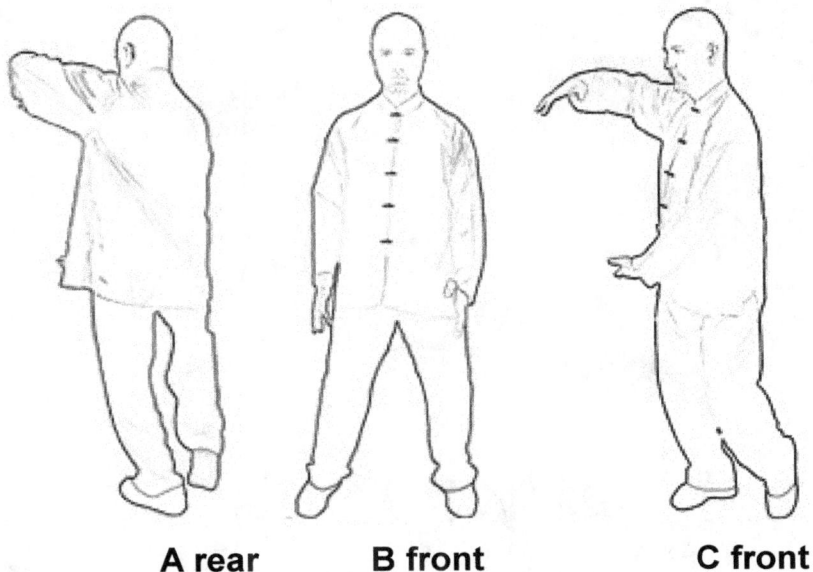

A rear   **B front**   **C front**

A   Bending from elbow, <u>left</u> arm sweeps over at shoulder height, palm facing down as <u>right</u> arm sweeps under, palm facing up (as if holding a large ball), stepping back onto the <u>right</u> toe.

B   Step to the <u>right</u> at about shoulder width, arms facing as if sweeping a ball down in front of the abdomen. Turning the <u>left</u> toe, face the front, feet parallel.

C   Move body weight over your <u>left</u> leg turning right toe out 45°, in the same way as previous movements, but on the opposite side. <u>Right</u> arm sweeps over and <u>left</u> arm sweeps under, palms facing as if holding a ball, at the same time moving body weight 100% over <u>right</u> leg, stepping up on <u>left</u> toe.

Section 6e

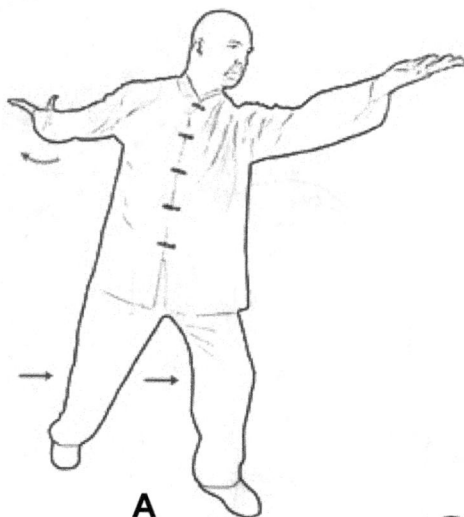

A

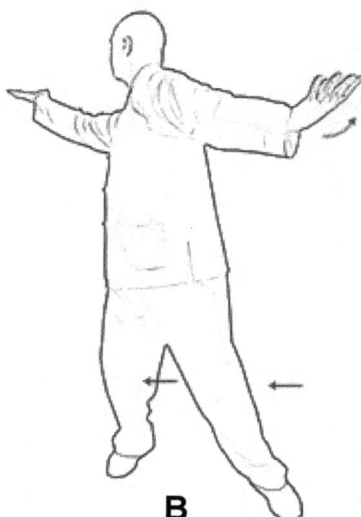

B

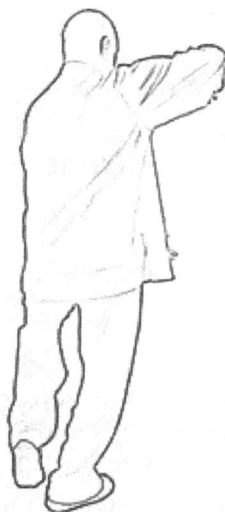

C rear

A Stepping forward with <u>left</u> leg, <u>left</u> arm sweeps forward palm facing up as <u>right</u> arm sweeps back palm facing up.

B As with previous movement, move back and forward three times, as a fire ball rolls from one palm across shoulders to other palm, twisting the arms and turning the palms to stretch the Heart and Small Intestine channel, bringing warmth to the heart and chest.

C Finish with 100% body weight over <u>right</u> leg, looking back, <u>right</u> arm sweeps over at shoulder height, palm facing down as <u>left</u> arm sweeps under, palm facing up (holding a large ball)

Section 6f

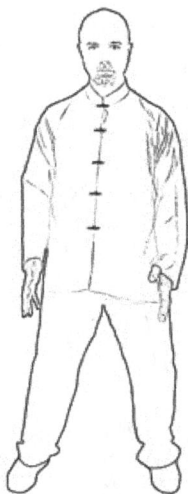

A

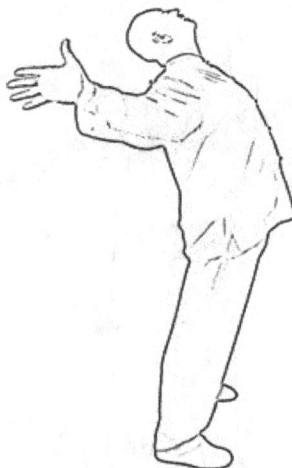

B side

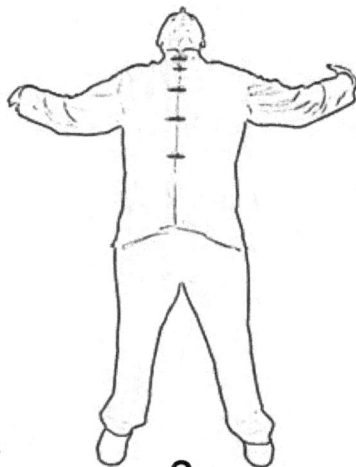

C

A Step to the <u>left</u> at about shoulder width, arms facing as if sweeping a ball down in front of the abdomen. Turn the <u>right</u> toe to face the front, feet parallel. Hold both arms to the side of body.

B Raise arms, extending them out at shoulder height. Lean back, opening the chest, fingers pulling back, extending the <u>middle finger</u> (Pericardium channel), and moving body to an upright position.

C Leaning back again, opening the chest, palms up extending the <u>little finger</u> back (Heart channel), move body to upright position.

Section 6g

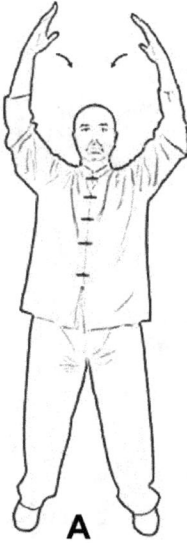

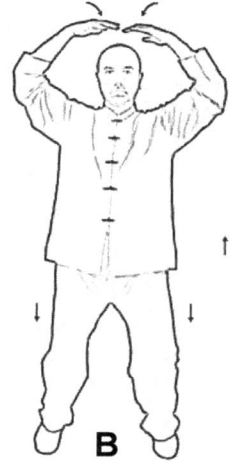

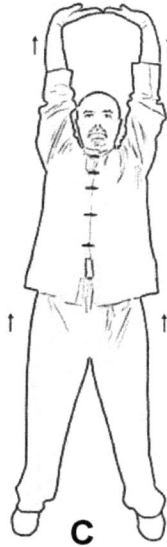

A, B Arms reach up into the sky gathering heavenly Qi to top of head (Bai Hui) with awareness down to Small Intestine.

C Turn palms up, fingers pointing towards each other, push to the sky, stretching heart and small intestine channels on outside of arms, then lift heels off ground, stretch.

Section 6h

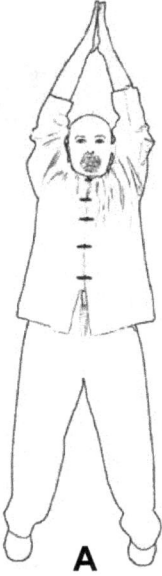

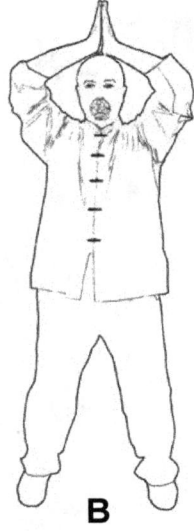

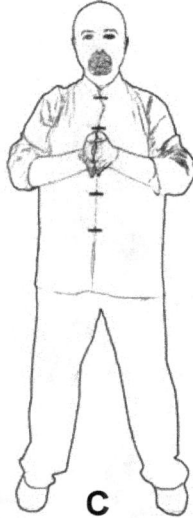

A, B, Return heels to the ground, palms together moving heavenly Qi
C into hands, bring hands to top of head (Bai Hui point), down to
the middle of the chest guiding heavenly Qi into the heart. Palms
turned down, fingers pointing down.

Section 6i

A

B

C side

D side

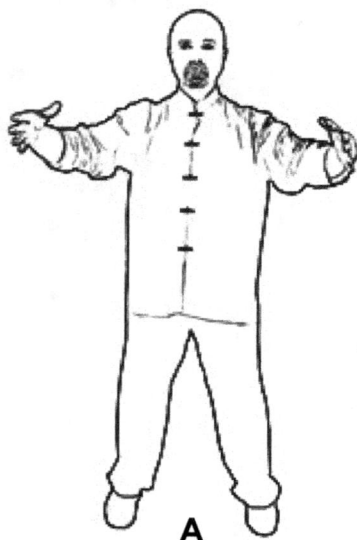

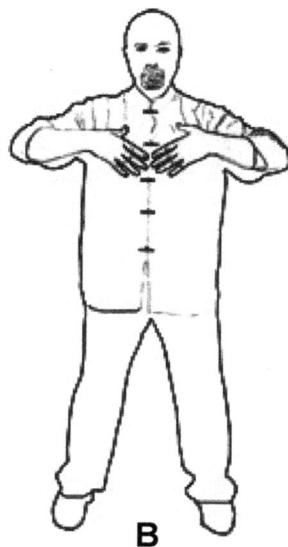

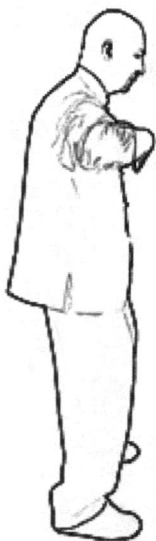

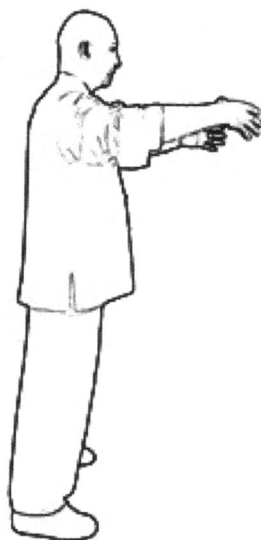

A, B, Elbows held high, moving hands in and away from heart three
C, D times. Breathing out as hands move away from heart, allow stale
Qi out and breathing in, hands move towards heart, allowing fresh
Qi in.

Section 6j

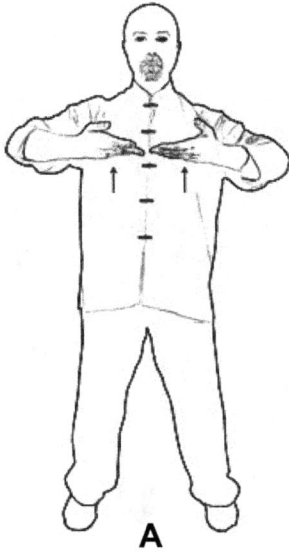

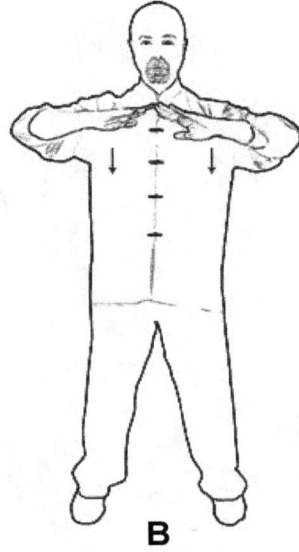

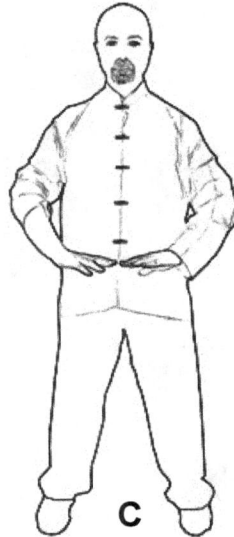

A Turn palms up, lifting to upper chest height, letting Jade Nectar (saliva) flow in the mouth as you think of the tip of the tongue.

B Turn palms to face ground and swallow Jade Nectar while slowly guiding hands and Jade Nectar to Dan Tian.

C Separate hands at Dan Tian, fingers pointing to ground.

Finish with closing movement

(See instructions page 30)

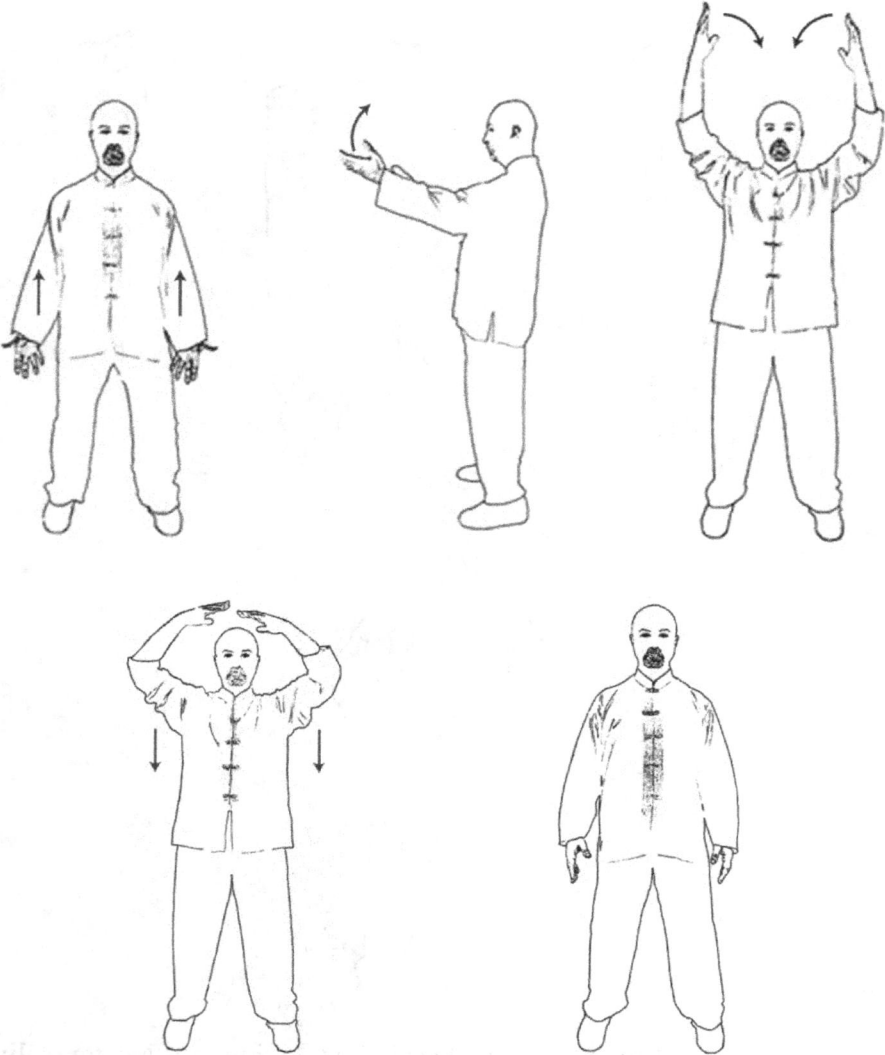

Complete this section again on the other side, starting with the left leg forward.

Repeat 3 times to both sides.

Hands on Dan Tian

The final section – meditation

Find a quiet, peaceful spot where you won't be disturbed. Either sit on a cushion or a chair, or lie down. Just relax, follow and watch the breath, staying in this position for at least 20 minutes. Allow your Qi to become clear and stable. As Dr Xu often says, "Nothingness is the best prescription".

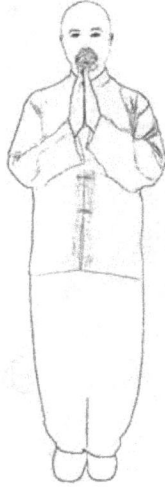

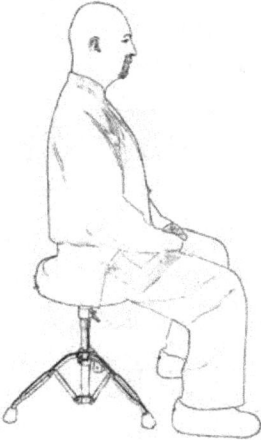

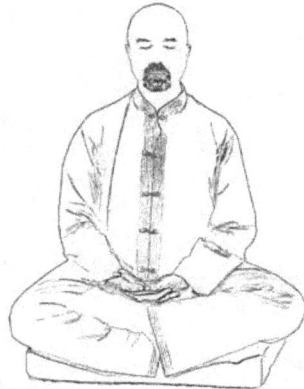

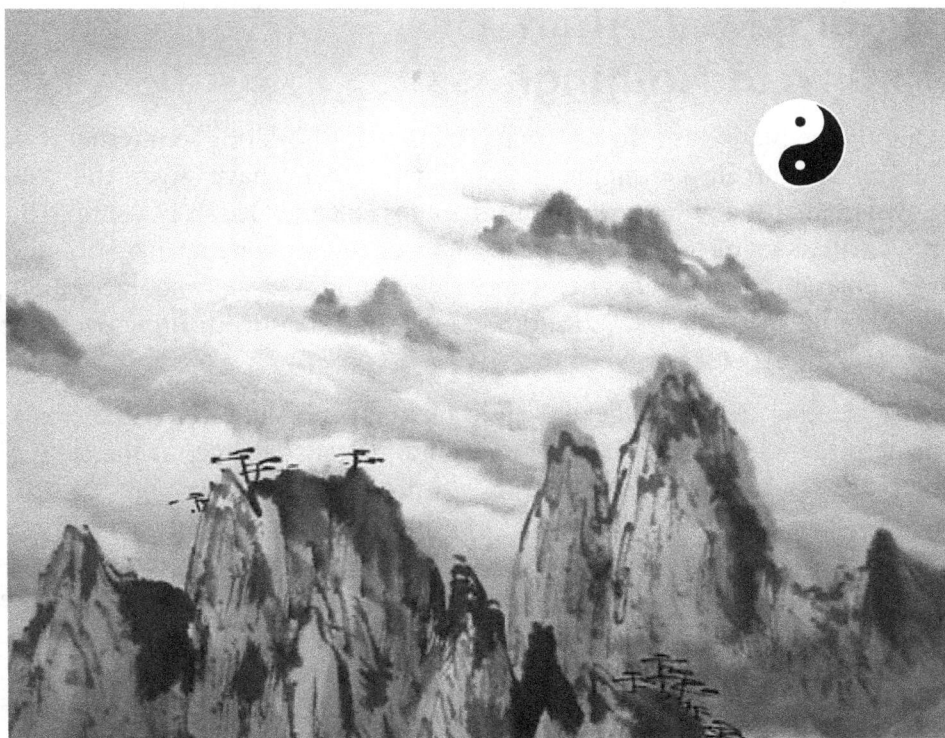

Chapter 11

Qigong Meditation
Return to Nothingness

Restoring Natural Harmony

Qigong Meditation – Return to Nothingness

Qigong meditation is also known as Nei Gong, translating to internal work or skill. Return to Nothingness is the name that I have given the lying down meditation practice that was given to me by Dr Xu. It is a simple but powerful technique. Dr Xu would often talk about its benefits in our training sessions with other Qigong teachers in Beijing. With his encouragement, the Qigong Meditation CD, Return to Nothingness, specifically devoted to this technique, was produced in 2006.

Most healing traditions have a style of lying meditation and their basic principles are similar. When we enter into a realised state, or the state of nothingness, in deep meditation, the Qi flows smoothly through the body as if we are tuning ourselves in to harmonise with the universe. In this state, significant healing can occur. These lying methods are also known as sleeping meditation or sleeping Qigong. If we consciously practise while we are lying in bed for about ten minutes before sleep, the Qi will continue to flow and we can continue practising Qigong while we sleep. Also, when awaking in the morning, we can return to the nothingness for a few minutes before getting up, allowing the Qi to continue flowing.

When I began to develop this practice I observed what I was doing when I was going to sleep and noted that the three main Qigong principles continued to apply – regulating the **posture** (relaxing the body), regulating the **breath** and regulating the **mind**. Firstly, it is necessary to relax and allow physical and emotional tension which has built up during the day to be released.

This practice is beneficial on its own or used in conjunction with Guigen Qigong. The technique can also be used for a sitting or standing meditation.

Preparation and practice

This meditation practice will help strengthen and increase your life force, or Qi energy. It's best done at night, lying on your bed, leading into a deep sleep, or when you have a few hours to rest during the day.

An important tip: when awakening in the morning or after practice, return to the nothingness for a few minutes before getting up.

To begin, lie down in a comfortable position either on your back or on your side.

Keeping your back straight, allow your awareness to travel up your spine – one vertebra at a time.

Try to release any tension in your body.

Just relax.

Allow your awareness to scan down your body, from your head down to your feet, like a wave dissolving any tension in your body.

Take your time . . . just relax.

Now, start to become aware of your breath.

Gently breathe in and out through your nose.

Let your breath become smooth and even.

Let your mind relax.

Allow the mind to follow the breath.

As you breathe in, the abdomen gently expands and as you let the breath out, the abdomen gently contracts.

Observe the flow of Qi to the Dan Tian, the energy centre at your lower abdomen, just below your navel.

Take your time, relax and feel.

Now, with each out breath, consciously allow your Qi to disperse from the Dan Tian, out through your whole body.

In all directions, allow your Qi to disperse throughout your whole body.

Through every cell, follow the Qi.

Relax and feel.

Now with each out breath, consciously allow your Qi to disperse further; now, beyond your body, out to the edge of the sheets or the mat you are lying on.

In all directions, like a large bubble or a spiraling galaxy, expanding out from your Dan Tian,

In all directions follow the Qi.

Relax and feel.

Allow your Qi to disperse out further,

Out to the mountains . . . towards the horizon,

Up into the clouds, and high above the earth . . . in all directions.

As you merge with the universe,

Return to Nothingness….. Nothingness….. Nothingness…...

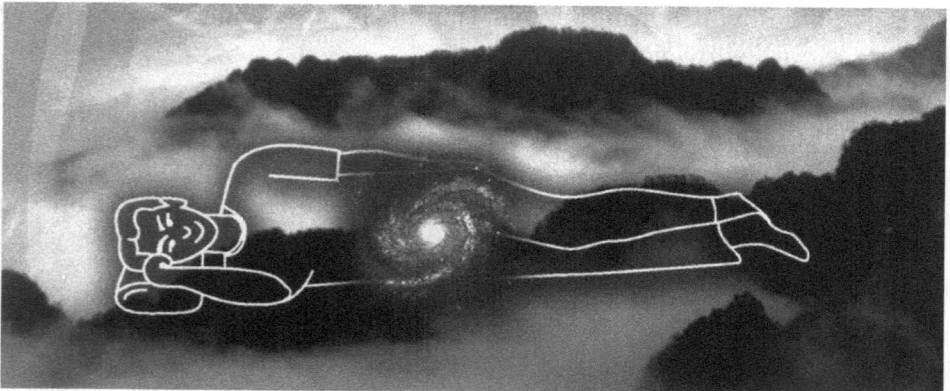

Meditation Points

1	命門	**Ming Men** Door to Life
2	玉枕	**Yu Zhen** Jade Pillow
3	百會	**Bai Hui** Hundred Points Converge
4	上丹田	**Upper Dan Tian** Upper Centre of Energy
5	中丹田	**Middle Dan Tian** Middle centre of Energy
6	丹田	**Dan Tian** Centre of Energy
7	會陰	**Hui Yin** Convergence of Yin Energy
8	長強	**Chang Qiang** End of Spine
9	涌泉	**Yong Chuan** Gushing Spring
10	勞宮	**Lao Gong** Palace of Labour

Diagram of the energy points around the body English, Chinese and Chinese characters

This is not a medical device and should not be used to replace any existing treatment, always check with your health provider if uncertain

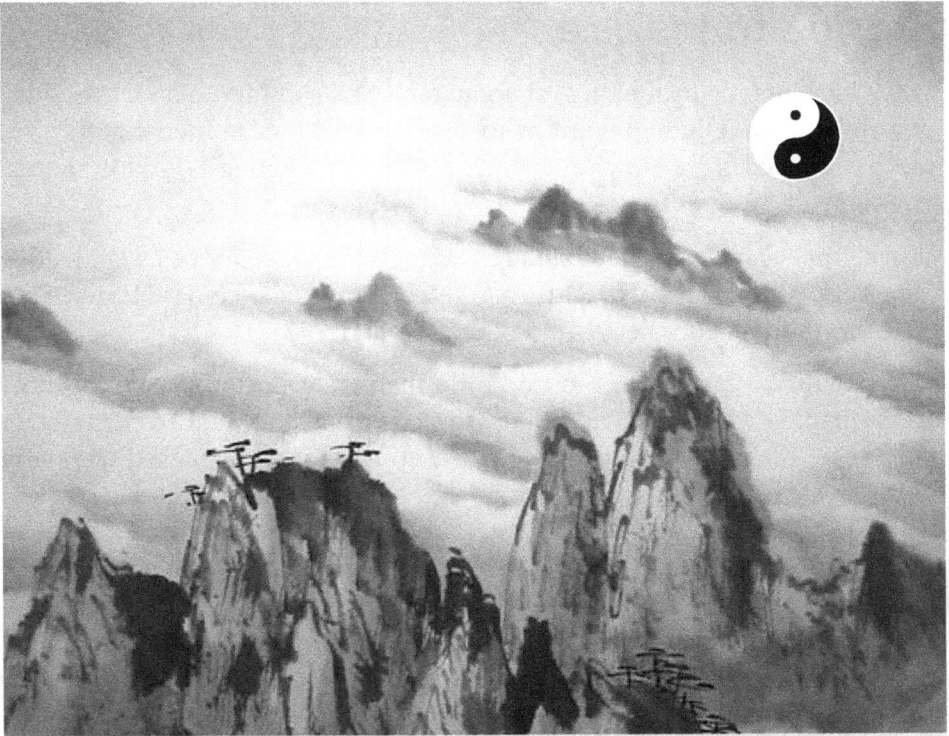

Chapter 12

Stories to Inspire

Restoring Natural Harmony

Stories to Inspire

I have been practising Qigong for about ten years and I try to do it every day as well as yoga. Qigong is linked to Traditional Chinese Medicine (TCM) and has existed for a very long time. So for me Qigong is giving me the benefit of TCM and the exercises, as well as the meditation.

Qigong makes me feel happy and relaxed, giving me inner peace and at the same time a lot of energy to affront the challenges of the day. It gives me more flexibility, better health and peace of mind.

I have realized that there is more to life than materialism. I have a deeper understanding of myself and others, the power of the mind over the body and the simple pleasures of everyday life. When I was diagnosed with very aggressive pre-cancerous cells in my right breast, I had radiotherapy and did Qigong. Qigong helped me a lot, giving me more energy and a positive attitude, helping me to recover more quickly. I have the privilege of being a Qigong instructor and the immense satisfaction of seeing the health of my students improve and hearing them at the end of the classes saying how relaxed and happy they are feeling, and how much they look forward to the next class. **Josette Libon, Victoria**

I have been practising Qigong for about eight years, 3-4 times per week. I started with Tai Chi for five years then after meeting Simon and participating in a China Tour I have cemented Qigong into my way of life.

My understanding of Qigong is that it is a meditative, gentle way of generating the energy flow through the meridians of my body, and a mental health massage that clears my thoughts. After practice I feel confident and happier. I am better able to face a busy day knowing that I am feeling aligned.

In my practice it is essential for me to be able to tune into my clients' energy. This is much easier when my energy channels are clear from Qigong practice. For me, Qigong is a safe state (place) to retreat to, for peace and calm.

I share my Qigong with others and they have also grown to love it. The combined energy of the group is beautiful. It is so nice to flow with others in peaceful harmony. I know my Qigong practice has also helped train my body so I can have a good postural stance for my big day of massaging, e.g., how to move with my whole energy flowing and not straining in one particular area. It also reminds me to connect to my breathing.
Shirley Alderson, NSW

Qigong has become a way of life for me, having practised it for 25 years. I still practice about 4-5 times a week. It restores my energy, balances my awareness of the 'now', and helps me maintain focus and stay peaceful within myself. It makes me feel that I am an important part of the community and that what I say and feel, matters. It makes me feel like an individual and I have found acceptance of self after a long search.

My mind likes the stillness. I particularly love the names of the movements. For me there is a connection with the name of the movement and when I practise I visualise the movement in my mind as I think how beautiful the name sounds. **Annie Oaff, NSW**

I have been practising Qigong once a week for at least eight or nine years. I was looking for something to give me gentle physical exercise, fluidity of movement and involvement at a spiritual level too.

Qigong lifts my energy, unblocks energy channels and lets the energy flow. I feel calm and invigorated at the same time. The meditation is also a very valuable part of the class. I feel more together and uplifted with more energy. It has helped me through some difficult times in my life.

Over the years I've learnt that my body needs nurturing and looking after and Qigong provides this gently, but also with strength. Practising Qigong helps me to focus better and to relax more easily. I have missed Qigong for a few months now due to study and travel commitments and I miss it! I find that the Monday evening class gives me a lift for most of the week. **Christiane LeCornu, NSW**

I have been practising Qigong since early 2009 and go to class once a week. It was the concept of 'energy' that I wanted to explore and how to work with shifting energy in and around the body.

I understand Qigong to be a way of bringing the body/mind system into a state of harmony which gives the human body/mind more 'ability' to make itself whole.

Qigong makes me feel as if my whole system is being exercised – physically and energetically. It leaves me feeling calm, peaceful and very content as if I have had a safe and gentle workout. The clearing of any energy blocks in my being gives me a peaceful feeling of wholeness, the ability to just 'be my essence'.

I've learnt that things are not always as they seem, that there are gentle, safe and nurturing ways to help you go through challenges in life and become more happy, calm and peaceful. I teach Dru Yoga which transforms energy through the heart chakra. I can feel the subtle effects of energy moving and clearing in my body/mind. I like Simon's style of teaching and his clear instructions, and that he comes from experience within himself. With gratitude. **Janet Beath, NSW**

I have been practising Qigong for four years between three to seven times a week. Initially I was practising and teaching Tai Chi but wanted a deeper understanding and experience of the underlying principles.

My understanding of Qigong is that it is movement which encourages the flow of energy through the natural pathways of the body, enhancing physical, emotional and spiritual health.

Qigong makes me feel balanced, centred, happier, content, compassionate, empathetic, safe and strong. It has improved my physical, mental, emotional and spiritual strength and the ability to help others. It gives me an increasing awareness of the oneness of humanity and the Universe, meditation being an integral part of Qigong.

I have practised different types of yoga and meditation for decades, however Qigong brings everything together for me. **Sandra Raggett, NSW**

I've been practising Qigong for nearly six years and try to do some practice everyday. When I was diagnosed with breast cancer I read about the benefits of Qigong for cancer patients and decided to investigate it.

My understanding of Qigong is that it's an ancient Taoist system of movement, breathing and meditation. Taoists believe that the Qi or life force, runs through all things and that stagnation or blockages of Qi in the body can cause illness. It can also enhance a sense of connectedness with internal and external energies, with nature and the spiritual dimension. Some people call it 'acupuncture without the needles'. Others say it is 'movement with breath awareness' or 'moving meditation'.

Qigong makes me feel calm, more relaxed and centred. It enhances my flexibility and boosts my energy. I believe regular Qigong practice has been significant in helping to control the effects of cancer. Not only is the practice enjoyable, it also provides a sense of control and of hope – great gifts if one has had a dire diagnosis. Qigong is safe, convenient, free and available to all! In my experience, Qigong can effectively be combined with a range of therapies and practices such as conventional cancer treatments, nutritional support, herbs, meditation and other energetic forms of healing.

After practising and meditating for three hours a day, over a ten-month period (combined with conventional medicine and other therapies), the cancer had totally retreated from my torso. Lungs, pelvis and chest were cancer free. I am convinced Qigong played a very important role in this.

I celebrated of course and let the intensive practice lapse and after some months the cancer reappeared in my bones. However, I could still feel optimistic about the future. Five years later (admittedly after many ups and downs) I'm still here and currently doing well. I certainly do not discount the impact of conventional medicine, which is crucial, but I am convinced Qigong can bring huge benefits to the practitioner.

I have learnt about the remarkable capacity of the body to heal itself given the right circumstances. I have a much stronger intuitive sense of what is happening within my own body, as well as a new sense of connection with the external, immaterial realm. **Marian Waller, NSW**

I have been practising Qigong for 16 years and currently practise every morning. I was dealing with severe depression and tried various forms of alternative therapy including Yoga and Qigong. Qigong makes me calm and helps me to understand that I must look at my whole body and outlook, not just concentrate on one part of myself.

It has improved my intestinal fortitude. I used to suffer from lots of stomach upsets but not any more. I am 71 years old and feel better than I did 10 years ago.

I have learnt that I am just a small part of the universe. My ego seems to have shrunk and I don't worry about things as I did before. I was lucky to be shown Qigong. Since I first began practising 15 years ago I have gone on a journey which becomes more and more interesting. It looks as if it will be with me for the rest of my life. My teachers have shared with me their experiences and insights generously. I have been fortunate to find these people while living in remote parts of Australia. Qigong is now a daily practice for me because, quite frankly, I feel better because of it. I have used DVDs and books which have proved useful, but I would recommend that the best way to learn is in a class. **Anonymous**

I have been practising Qigong for ten years now, normally about 3-4 times a week. After a life-threatening illness I was looking for a form of treatment to regain my health and strength and began practising Qigong.

It has been a great benefit to me. It charges me with energy and relieves my fatigue. My health has improved and I no longer suffer from depression. My body flexibility is also greatly enhanced.

During practice I attain a meditative state which is relaxing. My perceptions about what is important have changed and I feel more compassionate towards others. I have definitely reached a better balance in my life through Qigong practice. **Stephen Maddox, NSW**

I have been practising Qigong since January 2007 and attend a weekly class (approx two hours) and do 3-4 weekly sessions by myself. I started practising Qigong to improve my mind-body health as part of a centred approach to achieving a more satisfying work-life balance.

Having practised now for nearly three years I find I can cope much better with the stressful uncertainty of my work (rural GP). I think I'm more open to the needs of others because I'm more in touch with my inner self.

I have learnt that slowing down and breathing well with awareness can lead to happiness and efficiency! I find Qigong is great because it appears so simple and is easy for anyone to get started. The benefits begin without you being aware of them. As time goes by the meditative element of practice becomes stronger and even more rewarding. Qigong is a bridge to meditation and the benefits meditation brings. **Anonymous**

CDs – by Simon Blow

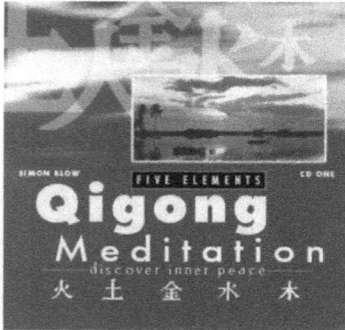

CD1: Five Elements Qigong Meditation

This CD is the perfect introduction to Qigong meditation (Neigong). **Track one** features a 30-minute heart-felt guided meditation to help bring love and light from the universe into your body. It harmonises the Five Elements – Fire, Earth, Metal, Water and Wood – with the corresponding organs of the body, respectively the heart, spleen, lungs, kidney and liver. This is one of the foundations of Chinese Qigong. Let Qigong Master Simon Blow help harmonise the elements of the universe with the energy of your body by using colour and positive images. **Track two** provides 30 minutes of relaxing music by inspiring composer Dale Nougher.

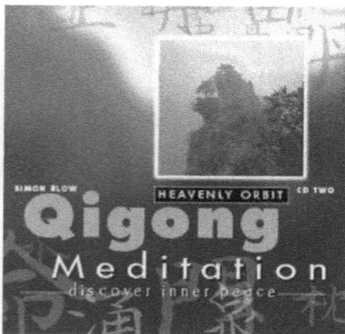

CD2: Heavenly Orbit Qigong Meditation

This CD is intended for the intermediate student. **Track one** takes you through a 30-minute guided meditation using your awareness to stimulate the energy centres around the body and open all the meridians. The circulation of Qi (Chi) around the Heavenly Orbit is one of the foundations of Chinese Qigong. The energy rising up the back 'Du' channel harmonises with the energy descending down the front 'Ren' channel, helping balance the energy of the body. Master Simon Blow guides you to open the energy centres of your own body to create harmony with the universe. **Track two** provides 30 minutes of relaxing music by Dale Nougher.

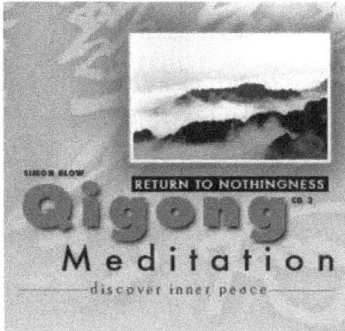

CD3: Return to Nothingness Qigong Meditation

This CD is intended for the advanced student and those wanting a healing night-practice. One of the aims of Qigong is to allow our internal energy (Qi) to harmonise with the external energy (Qi) allowing our consciousness to merge with the universe. When we enter into a deep sleep or meditation all the meridians start to open and much healing can take place. In this 20-minute guided meditation Simon Blow assists you in guiding your energy through your body and harmonising with the energy of the universe. Track two provides 30 minutes of healing music by Dale Nougher.

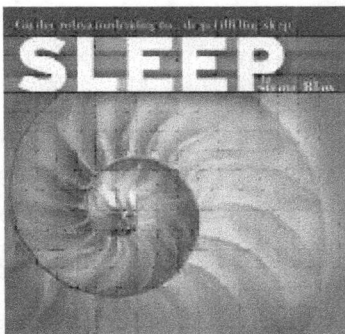

Sleep

Sleep is necessary to maintain life, alongside breathing, eating, drinking, and exercising of the mind and body. Without a good six to eight hours of sleep each night it can be hard to live a quality, balanced, fulfilling life. When we sleep it's a time to rest and rejuvenate the mind and body and to release the physical, mental and emotional stress that has built up during the day. This also helps uplift us spiritually.

It's a time to rest; it's time for a good night's sleep. Let Simon Blow's soothing voice, along with Dale Nougher's beautiful piano music and the natural sounds of the ocean, help guide you to release the tension of the day and enable you to enter a deep, fulfilling sleep.

Book/DVD sets – by Simon Blow

"About 18 months ago I started to practise Qigong as I knew that it would improve my health. I needed to do it regularly, ideally every day, but being in a rural area presented logistical problems. I discovered Simon's DVD and commenced daily practice. The great advantage for me was that I didn't have to travel to classes and could do them whenever I felt like it. Since that time I have noticed great improvement in my overall wellbeing. It has helped me to reinvent my clinical practice as a holistic massage practitioner. A number of my clients now have Simon's DVD and I feel this is helping them to both improve their health and well being, and to empower themselves." **Robin Godson-King (Holistic Massage Practitioner)**

(Each set contains a DVD plus a book that provides diagrams and instructions for the movements contained on the DVD. The book also includes interesting reading about the practice of Qigong as well as inspirational stories.)

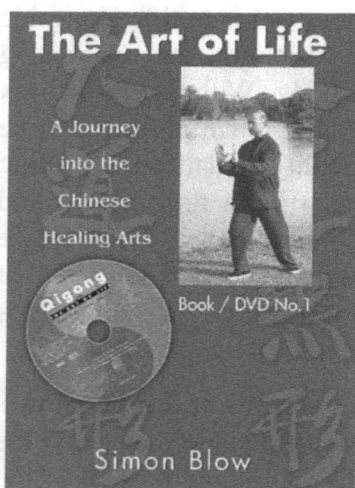

The Art of Life

'The Art of Life' presents the Qigong styles that were taught to me in Australia: the Taiji Qigong Shibashi, which I learned as an instructor with the Australian Academy of Tai Chi from 1990 to 1995; and the Ba Duan Jin standing form, commonly known as the Eight Pieces of Brocade, taught to me in 1996 by Sifu John Dolic in Sydney.

This is the perfect introduction to this ancient art and is suitable for new and continuing students of all ages. The book follows the DVD and contains three sections: **1. Warm up** – gentle movements loosen all the major joints of the body, lubricating the tendons and helping increase blood and energy circulation. It is beneficial for most arthritic conditions; **2. Ba Duan Jin or Eight Pieces of Brocade** – this is the best known and most widely practised form of Qigong throughout the world, also known as Daoist Yoga. The movements stretch all the major muscles, massage organs and open the meridians of the body; **3. Taiji Qigong Shibashi** – this popular practice is made up of eighteen flowing movements. The gentle movements harmonise the mind, body and breath. Total running time: 55 minutes.

"Tai Chi Qigong is a gentle way of exercising the whole body and provides long-term benefits. I recommend it to my patients as an effective way of improving muscle tone and joint mobility. Those who practise regularly have fewer problems with their muscles and joints and often report an increased sense of health and wellbeing. This is an excellent video with clear and simple instruction."
Roman Maslak. B.A. (Hons), D.O. Osteopath

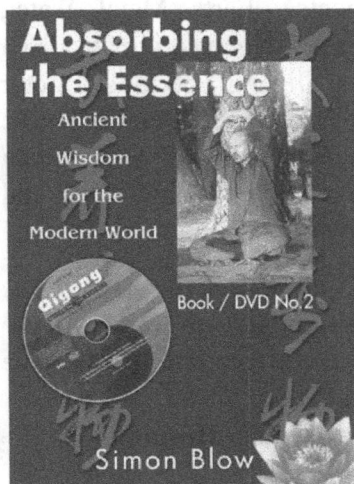

Absorbing the Essence

'Absorbing the Essence' comprises the Qigong cultivation techniques that were taught to me by Grand Master Zhong Yunlong in 1999 and 2000 at Wudangshan or Wudang Mountain. Wudang is one of the sacred Daoist Mountains of China and is renowned for the development of Taiji.

This DVD and book is for the intermediate student and for people with experience in meditation. It contains three sections: **1. Warm up** – the same as in The Art of Life DVD; **2. Wudang Longevity Qigong** – this sequence of gentle, flowing movements stimulates the Heavenly Orbit, absorbing the primordial energy from the environment and letting the negativity dissolve into the distance; **3. Sitting Ba Duan Jin** – this 30-minute sequence includes eight sections with exercises to stimulate different organs and meridians of the body. It is practised in a seated position on a chair or cushion – ideal for people who have discomfort whilst standing. These practices originated from the famous Purple Cloud Monastery at the sacred Wudang Mountain in China. Total running time: 60 minutes.

"Simon Blow of Australia has twice travelled (1999, 2000) to Mt Wudang Shan Daoist Wushu College to learn Taiji Hunyuan Zhuang (Longevity) Qigong and Badajin Nurturing Life Qigong and through his study has absorbed the essence of these teachings. Therefore, I specially grant Simon the authority to teach these, spreading the knowledge of these Qigong methods he has learnt at Mt Wudang to contribute to the wellbeing of the human race. May the Meritorious Deeds Be Infinite."
Grand Master Zhong Yunlong, Daoist Priest and Director,
Mt Wudang Shan Taoist Wushu College, China, September 24, 2000.

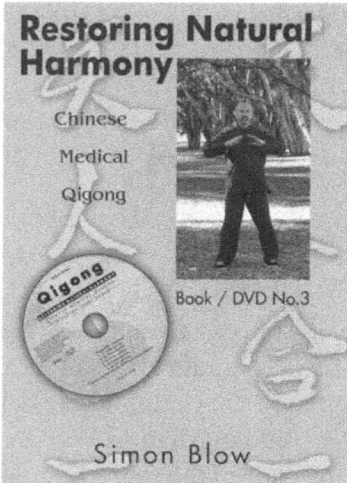

Restoring Natural Harmony

This DVD and book is for the advanced student or for the person wanting to learn specific Traditional Chinese Medicine self-healing exercises. Each section works on a different organ meridian system of the body – Spleen, Lungs, Kidney, Liver and Heart – which relate to the Five Elements – Earth, Metal, Water, Wood and Fire. Guigen Qigong originated from Dr Xu Hongtao, a Qigong Specialist Doctor from the Xiyuan Hospital in Beijing. These internal exercises help regulate the meridian system bringing harmony to mind, body and spirit. Total running time: 75 minutes.

"Simon Blow first visited our hospital in 2002. I was impressed with his knowledge and commitment to Qigong. He returned in 2004 to study Chinese Medical Qigong. Simon is a gifted teacher: he has the rare ability to inspire others and impart to them the healing benefits of Qigong."
Dr Xu Hongtao, Qigong and Tuina Department, Xiyuan Hospital Beijing, China.

"This DVD – the third by the impressively qualified Sydney-based Simon Blow – serves two purposes. Firstly, it is so attractively produced that the curious would surely be induced to investigate further. Secondly, for those already practising, it provides a mnemonic device much more useful than a series of still pictures." **Review by Adyar Bookshop, Sydney 2005.**

These are not medical devices and should not be used to replace any existing medical treatment. Always consult with your health provider if uncertain.

To order products or for more information on:

- Regular classes in Sydney for new and continuing students
- Workshops or if you would be interested in helping organise a workshop in your local area
- Residential Qigong and Meditation retreats
- China Qigong Study Tours for students and advanced training
- Talks, corporate classes, training and presentations
- Wholesale enquiries

Please contact:

Simon Blow
PO Box 446
Summer Hill, NSW 2130
Sydney Australia

Ph: +61 (0)2 9559 8153
Email: info@simonblowqigong.com
Web: **www.simonblowqigong.com**

CDs and Book/DVDs can be ordered online and shipped nationally and internationally.

Bibliography

Publications
Dechar, Lorie Eve. *Five Spirits*. New York: Lantern Books, 2006.

Liu Qingshan. *Chinese Fitness*. Massachusetts: YMAA Publication Centre, 1997.

Ni Hua-Ching. *Tao: The Subtle Universal Law and the Integral Way of Life* (2nd edn). California: Seven Star Communications Group, Inc., 1995.

Ni Hua-Ching. *Esoteric Tao Teh Ching*. California: Seven Star Communications Group, Inc., 1992.

Yang, Jwing-Ming. *The Root of Chinese Gigong*, Massachusetts: YMAA Publication Centre, 1997.

Websites
Suite 101: Chinese Medicine. **http://chinese-medicine.suite101.com/ article.cfm/tcm_and_the_internal_organs**

Acupuncture Online, by Meredith St John. **www.acupuncture-online. com/tradition3.htm**

Meridian Diagrams
Original meridian diagrams sourced from:
Wu Changguo. *Basic Theory of Traditional Chinese Medicine*. China: Publishing House of Shanghai University of Traditional Chinese Medicine.

www.ingramcontent.com/pod-product-compliance
Lightning Source LLC
Chambersburg PA
CBHW070806290326
41931CB00011BA/2149